A GUILTY VICTIM

Recovering Creativity after Trauma and Abuse

Toby Ingham

with illustrations by William Smith

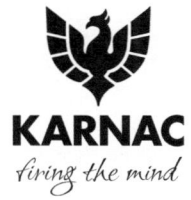

KARNAC

firing the mind

First published in 2025 by
Karnac Books Limited
62 Bucknell Road
Bicester
Oxfordshire OX26 2DS

British Library Cataloguing in Publication Data

A C.I.P. for this book is available from the British Library

ISBN: 978-1-80013-306-8 (paperback)
ISBN: 978-1-80013-340-2 (e-book)
ISBN: 978-1-80013-341-9 (PDF)

Typeset by vPrompt eServices Pvt Ltd, India

www.firingthemind.com

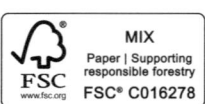

Karnac Books is committed to a sustainable future for our business, our readers, and our planet. This book is made from Forest Stewardship Council® certified paper.

A GUILTY VICTIM

'To restore the human subject at the centre—the suffering, afflicted, fighting, human subject, we must deepen the case history to a narrative or tale.'

—Oliver Sacks, *The Man Who Mistook His Wife for a Hat*, 1985

'I see it differently now, but back then I was in an impossible situation and I suppose I just went along with him. He was a priest, priests ran the school and you did what they said. He said if I came with him he'd let me smoke in his room. I only wanted tobacco.'

—William Smith, 2018

About the author

Toby Ingham is a UK-based psychotherapist and supervisor and a former clinical director of South Bucks Counselling. His writing has been commended in the *British Journal of Psychotherapy*.

Acknowledgements

I would like to acknowledge and thank the people who have helped me think through aspects of my work during the writing of this book. First, my profound gratitude to William Smith, without whom none of this would have been possible.

Thank you to the team at Karnac: Kate Pearce, Anita Mason, and Nick Downing. Thanks are also due to David Henderson, Loraine McSherry, Nick Smith, and to my colleagues at The Association of Independent Psychotherapists. To colleagues who heard presentations of early clinical material: Donald Kalsched, and West Midlands Institute of Psychotherapy, Middlesex University Centre for Psychoanalysis, South Bucks Counselling, and Riverside Counselling Service. Thanks to friends who read and commented on early drafts: Alastair Wheelhouse, Carl Dines, Charles Bainbridge, Dylan Ward, Julia Appleton, Samantha Tu, Simon Russell, Mahmood Al Sa Bari, Rowan Hisayo Buchanan and colleagues at Faber & Faber Academy, Stephen Carver at The Literary Consultancy, and Sam Jordison at Jericho Writers.

To Maria, Harry, and Alice, thank you for everything.

Introduction

This is a true story of a man's struggle in psychotherapy to free himself from a dangerous self-destructive mindset. I've given him a pseudonym, William Smith, to protect his identity, but this account has been written with his full consent.

When I first met William, he was fifty-four years old and battling with feelings of worthlessness and depression. He had been suicidal at earlier periods in his life and came to see me because he had concerns that those feelings were returning. We worked together for several years and in that time we began to see how he had internalised a critical and aggressive attitude which picked on and bullied what might be thought of as his true self. Any attempt to express himself creatively was met with fierce prohibition. William could do things for other people but not for himself. Towards the end of our work William created a set of pictures, a timeline of his life, and he suggested that I write text to go with the pictures. This book is that text.

Over the course of a long period of psychotherapy a great deal of information is gathered both about a client's life and experiences, and about the process of working together to uncover those details. Information emerges organically, piecemeal, and that can create a problem of how to organise it. Writing an account of the work and basing it around William's illustrated timeline, provided a framework and solved a problem of how to structure this account.

The central idea of the book is that we suffer not because there is something wrong with us, but because of things that have happened to us. The problem is we often lose sight of those things, or don't pay them enough attention.

Case studies are a valuable way of showing what happens in psychotherapy. By necessity they are often extracts from therapy rather than a full account, and they are often created around composite individuals because of the need to protect a client's identity. It is unusual to have the opportunity to write a case study with a client's permission and approval. I felt that if this was to be written up, then it should be aimed at as wide a readership as possible. A book for general readers, not just for academics, psychotherapists, and counsellors but for people who might be able to relate to the story and might be inspired to investigate their own lives and timelines further. I didn't want this to be a technical book, and I have intentionally avoided jargon and professional explanations and tried instead to show the way the process of psychotherapy unfolds in a series of ordinary if unusual conversations. Throughout, I have tried to keep William's story at the fore.

Psychotherapy isn't about saying clever things or making clever interpretations. It's about being reliable and predictable and trying to find a way to be with someone so that they might be able to settle, their defences lower, and their emotional stability improve. Something has brought the client to psychotherapy; we can never be entirely sure where that impulse began, but we can try to nurture it and see where it might be trying to go.

Among other things, I hope that this book will contribute to the way people think about early trauma, boarding school syndrome, and grooming. Grooming isn't the whole of this story, but it is part of it. Also, that it might contribute to an understanding of the creative dimension of psychotherapy.

A Guilty Victim is told in seven parts and is written in the form of flashback dramatisations interspersed with extracts from psychotherapy. William's timeline pictures are included in Part V. The book begins with a series of four psychotherapy sessions which illustrate how trust began to develop between us. Initially things were touch and go, but gradually the defences that had built up within him, and which kept William apart from his creativity, started to soften and he was able to say more about what he had been through. This led us to the story of his early childhood, and to a set of traumatic experiences that left him, as a schoolboy, vulnerable to the attention of a paedophile priest. Vulnerability is one of the key traits that predators pick up on.

Though the psyche may have been ravaged by toxic experiences, it still possesses the capacity to develop, recover, and to grow, and so go on to form new and healthy psychological adaptations. Although this is William's story, it might be every person's story too.

I gave William a pseudonym, William Smith, and I decided the narrative worked better if I gave myself one too, so in the text any reference to Julian Tate is a reference to me. I have written this account from my session notes. William has seen and reviewed every word.

Part I

Psychotherapy begins

Chapter 1

When someone asks me what psychotherapy is, I say this: psychotherapy is a unique form of conversation, it deepens and unfolds over time. Speaking about emotional pain can feel risky, but discovering the courage to put your experiences into words can be the start of developing insight and self-confidence. Over time, as the conversations develop, profound worries and anxieties can gradually take on more ordinary proportions. But of course, at the start, none of this can be taken for granted.

Before William came to see me we'd spoken once on the phone and he'd told me that he was looking to speak about his persistent low mood. At that time I worked from a room in my garden, it was away from the house and had its own parking area which made it discreet and private. I remember William arrived on time, that he delayed before getting out of his car and then stood for a moment looking around, he was a tall and imposing man. When I opened the door to meet him, he seemed apprehensive and took his time organising himself before coming in. I guessed he was about fifty, about my age.

Watching as he wrestled his green jacket off, I pointed to a hook on the wall.

'It's fine,' said William, flattening the jacket against the bulk of his stomach and glancing around the room. I kept the furniture simple, two chairs, the one nearest the door for my clients so they wouldn't feel trapped, a couch, a few pictures of landscapes, and a print of Van Gogh's *Room at Arles*. From his body language I had the impression that William might not be staying long.

I told him this was a confidential conversation, and that we had fifty minutes to think about what had brought him, after that a short silence ensued.

'Should I start?' William asked.

'Sure,' I said—I try to avoid leading conversations.

He leant forward, elbows pressed into his thighs, most of his jacket disappearing. I noticed a hint of aftershave, something lemony.

'I'm not sure where to start, I've been trying not to think about it, but I'm unhappy, depressed, self-critical, I've never been anything else.' He raised his eyes and creases spread across his forehead. 'It's the endless negative thinking, any sense of personal achievement triggers feelings of worthlessness in me, stops me doing things, didn't want me coming today. And it's old, it started at school. I was unhappy there and I found a way of fitting in by emulating some other boys.'

'Emulating,' I said. The word caught my attention.

'Yes, I found a way of fitting in by emulating them, I was good at sport. I wasn't particularly interested but it gave me a way in. At school if you're good at sport you fit in, so I copied other boys, emulated them, and it worked, for a while, but then we fell out and everything changed. When I left school I started drinking and I've never stopped. I need to get on top of the anxiety, the self-doubt, the endless critical monologue, the hyper-vigilance and the destructive drinking.' He leant his head back against the padding of the chair. 'I wasn't sure if I'd tell you all that.'

'You said you've been trying not to think about it.'

'I worried that if I thought about it too much I wouldn't come. I need to find a way out of this, there are things I want to do.'

'What kind of things?'

'Oh …' William gave a vague hand gesture, I noticed a silver ring on his right hand. A hint of a smile came and went, perhaps he sensed encouragement. 'Stop beating myself up for one, allow myself the freedom to follow my ideas, creative ideas.'

I asked him if he'd been in therapy before.

'I've seen a couple of people over the years, it's never worked, but I need to change.' Then after a pause he added 'Why did you ask about emulating?'

His question was quick, direct, I thought of him having to emulate to fit in, and the pair of us, meeting for the first time, how were we supposed to fit together?

'I wondered where you'd learnt to emulate,' I said.

William didn't seem to care for my reply.

'I haven't come here because of where I learnt to emulate. I'm here because I beat myself up.'

'Yes I see that,' I said, aware that the conversation had acquired a critical quality.

William drummed his fingers on the pale veneered arm of the chair, his left hand moved across his jacket. I thought he might be about to get up and leave. I noticed his pale blue eyes fix on the Van Gogh.

'Why have you got that picture in here?'

'You don't think it should be here?'

'No.'

'What don't you like about it?' I asked. I felt put on the spot but tried not to be defensive.

'The picture is fine, it's rather moving, do you know the room he's painted?' I did, but I kept that to myself. 'That's his bedroom at Arles isn't it, the psychiatric hospital,' said William. 'I like the picture. I just wonder why it's here?'

Thinking how best to reply I said, 'I think it mirrors this room, in a way.' He seemed to acknowledge there was something in that and leant back, the chair reclining with him. I felt myself relax a little. 'But you don't think it should be here?' I said, interested to find out more about what he didn't like. William looked unsure of whether to say any more, but then sat up.

'Van Gogh suffered. You might like the picture, but people who suffer might not want to look at it, all the strange perspectives, it might remind them of misery.' I found myself thinking he was making a good point, but almost immediately he seemed to backtrack. 'I'm sorry,' he said, 'I don't mean to be rude.'

'I don't know if you're being rude, I think you're making a point, thinking about who you're with, what sort of therapist puts Van Gogh's room on his wall?' I realised as I said it that I wasn't sure myself. William swivelled in his chair and closed his eyes, from outside the room I heard bird song and the murmur of traffic.

'I like your shed, I'm sorry, I mean office, I feel I'm being rude again.'

'It is a kind of shed,' I said, though I was still thinking about the painting and wondered if I'd made a mistake putting it there, but it felt like we were on friendlier ground and I decided not to pursue it further for now.

'No,' said William, 'it's nicer than that, it's a very nice shed. I was thinking I'd come for a few appointments, just to see what it's like, this time works for me, could we keep this time for the next few weeks?'

I checked my diary.

'Yes,' I said, 'this time is fine.'

'How do you like to be paid?' asked William, his wallet appearing from his coat pocket. I told him I would give him a bill at the end of the month.

'That's rather trusting,' said William, 'the last person wanted cash each time.'

After William left, I remember leaning back against the desk thinking we'd only just avoided everything falling apart at the start. I wondered if that was how his previous therapies had gone and I recalled him saying that his self-critical side didn't want him coming today, it made me think of the things that got in the way of his creative ideas.

First sessions often give indications of what is to come and William had made an impression on me, the way the mood changed, warm then cold then warm again. I knew that you couldn't make people come to psychotherapy, that something in William had to hook into something in the therapy, and I felt some sympathy for him, this quick-witted man who could suddenly turn on himself, or me, with his direct questions, and I felt uneasy about the picture. Had someone come who would challenge everything about my setup? Had I put an image of suffering, self-harm, and suicide on the wall? I wondered if everyone who came thought the same? What to do? Removing it would be reactive, for better or worse it would have to stay.

Chapter 2

When the weather turned I would leave my house early to check on the heating before clients arrived. Sometimes on stormy days when I opened the door the linen curtains would billow out at me like melodramatic ghosts. I often wished I had a room in the house. Firing up the gas heater, I checked my diary and read through my notes. I have always been a prolific note-taker and in the ten-minute breaks between clients I write up sessions from memory: it's a habit developed during years of training that I've never given up, part conscientious, part driven by a guilt complex that pushed me to keep records, to be accountable. Sometimes I ended up writing so fast that I struggled to decipher them later.

William and I had now been working together for several months. During that time he had been punctual and never missed a session, but he was cagey, and often found it hard to trust me. I was interested in the history of his low mood, but whenever I tried to find out more he'd shut my questions down and tell me that I was missing the point.

———•———

'I'm not sure I'm getting my point across,' said William. He bit his lip, took a breath, then tried again. 'All the time I am scanning for threats and,' he pointed hard at me making sure the emphasis wasn't being missed, then seemed to catch himself and pressed his hand back into his green jacket pocket. 'Sorry, but I must keep it all secret. My family mustn't worry.'

'This is serious,' I said, trying to demonstrate by my tone that he might not be worrying me.

William grunted.

I became aware again of the gale blowing outside, of the rain lashing at the room, shaking the cedar roof tiles and spilling over the gutter. One of the curtains swayed as if by itself, the wind having found its way in.

'I don't know how long I am going to come here, but I want to try and tell you how it is. I'm scanning all the time, trying to spot everything, other people can have nice things, not me. You're ok to talk to, but I don't know if this does anything for me. Every morning it's the same voice, "I'm a piece of shit. I drink too much." It doesn't make any sense, I might not have drunk the night before, that doesn't matter, whatever I've done, the aggressive thoughts are at me, telling me I'm worthless.'

A small branch, broken off by the wind, clattered on the roof, interrupting him. William looked up, I winced, embarrassed that we were sitting in this lightweight garden shed.

'Sometimes the sneer is even worse when I haven't been drinking, it doesn't make any sense. In the morning, when I go to the bathroom, when I shave, it's there.' William puffed out his lips, sighed, closed his eyes, 'anyway, that's the point.' He put his hand down, opened his eyes, 'were you going to say something?'

'I was thinking about the way that voice reacts to you coming here. It sounds like these sessions stay on your mind during the week.'

'What? Do you think that's a good sign?'

'I'm not sure,' I said, trying to add a moderating tone to our conversation, 'but it caught my attention.' Outside the rain eased up a bit, the tension seemed to lessen a degree, perhaps two. I had become more used to his directness and tried to amplify my point, 'and it seems worse when you have a spontaneous thought.'

'That's also true,' said William, becoming more engaged, 'anything spontaneous sets it off,' he made a sort of snort laugh. 'Really I could be talking about my father. My father loved the golf club and his golf club cronies, horrible bigoted people. A nasty bunch of misogynists, failed marriages and low handicaps. He liked to joke that he once had three children under five, the same as his handicap.' He gave me a measured look. 'Do you play golf?' Before I could think to reply, William said, 'I don't like golf clubs. Anyway, don't tell me. I sometimes played golf with my father and his friends, they put everyone and everything down.'

'You haven't said much about your birth family.'

'I suppose I just started talking when I first came here,' said William. 'My mother and father are still married, to each other, sorry that's another one of my father's jokes. I have an older brother and sister, then there's me, then there's a gap to my younger sister.'

'How big is the gap?'

'What?'

'What are the age differences between you and your siblings?'

'My elder brother and sister and I are the three under-fives. Then there's a gap, eight years, to my sister.'

'Do you know why there was a gap like that?'

'Does it matter?'

'I don't know,' I said, 'that was why I was asking.' William looked at his hands, tapping his knuckles together.

'Maybe they wanted a break after me.' He swivelled his chair and looked out of the window. 'I don't know. I've not thought about it.'

'When you first came here you told me about falling out with friends at school, but I think this is part of an older story.' William turned back to me.

'I want to stop what's going on now, I've always linked it to events at school. I didn't see any reason to bring up anything else.'

'I wondered if learning to emulate, to copy, was older than that?'

'I don't think so,' said William.

'I know you don't think so,' I said, holding to my line.

'You think that something was going on before I went to school?'

'Well, I wondered about your early life.'

William pushed back in his chair, retreating into himself. I noticed him glance at the Van Gogh, his right knee tapping a fast rhythm all by itself. He shot a glance at the small objects on my desk, a small bronze owl and a bust of Odysseus, then looked past them and out at the garden.

We both watched the olive tree being blown about, I could feel the cabin brace against the wind.

'You're really out in the weather here.'

'You could say so,' I said, 'but we know there is more to you than this hypervigilance.'

'How do we know that?' William asked.

'We know how much you care for your family. When it comes to your wife and children nothing is too much.'

'But that's part of the set-up, I can do things for other people.' He swivelled his chair towards the window. 'Last year I had to write a legal letter, for work. I spent hours over it and became more and more immersed in the details of what I was writing. And at some point I realised that the critical soundtrack had stopped, and there was no negative thinking. It was temporary, it came back, but for those hours I was free of it. When I leave here, after one of our conversations, I sometimes feel better, lighter, then I get in my car and almost immediately I,' he broke off searching for a word, 'I flip, and all the good feeling is gone. There is just that voice saying I'm a piece of shit. It'll be waiting for me in the car. I'll look in the mirror and it will look back at me, and I'll go and buy cider and gin on my way home and then I'll drink and attack myself.' He shrugged and started to gather his things, leant forward in his chair and stood. 'I don't know why, but I'm not able to keep good feelings.'

I didn't think it was the right time to say anything else and I stood by my chair as William pulled the door shut behind him, careful not to catch the curtains, he had learnt the knack of them.

I watched his car edge out of the driveway, and I thought of disappointments, of the ghosts of disagreements people had come to have with me, issues I'd become embroiled in. People who had come often for more obscure reasons than could be quickly understood, but who in the end had lost heart or patience with the process and abandoned the idea.

William's ghosts waited in his car, pooled in his rear-view mirror, waiting to gang up on him. They thought he was making a mistake talking about all this. Like all the other mistaken attempts he'd made.

'Get yourself a drink,' they hissed, over the click of the indicator. 'And don't start telling him any of that.'

I found out later that when he left his sessions he would drive to different off-licences, always trying to find ones he'd not been to before.

For change to happen, the problem that has brought the client needs to come to be felt to be active within the therapeutic relationship so that it can be worked on between therapist and client. You can't make that happen on demand, a psychotherapist isn't there to force things, but together you might be able to work towards it.

The way I understood it, William thought that his problems related to his destructive mindset, low mood, and drinking and he saw this as linked to events that happened at school, the falling out. While I could see this was true, I still wondered about the word 'emulating', it made me wonder about him having already learnt to do something, to copy, to cover things up before he went to boarding school. He was resistant to my suggestions, and I was aware that pushing my ideas could easily cause him to stop coming, after all he'd stopped therapy in the past.

I now had a better grasp of the relationships in his family, and I wondered about the eight-year gap between him and his younger sister. I had a sense of his father, his anger, but very little idea about his mother, he'd said almost nothing about her.

He had made the point that things were worse for him when he had time on his hands, which made me think of him having been left waiting for too long, but I hadn't learnt anything more about that. Psychotherapy requires patience, being able to wait and tolerate not knowing things. I focused on trying to keep things predictable so that William might come to settle.

Chapter 3

William missed his next session. He later told me he 'got stuck into his work, thought this will do, no more navel gazing, fuck that. Fuck stupid therapy woke bullshit.' He said his father would have approved.

While his wife, Meg, was at work he holed up in his office. He tried to concentrate on his accounts, VAT, making money, and took his mood out on cold callers. He forced himself to focus, move on, get on with his life, do some exercise, lose some weight, get on with a photography project. It was down to him to sort himself out.

I sent him an email. He ignored it.

I found out later that he'd started drinking more, in secret, sipping gin from the bottle when he was alone in the kitchen, trying to self-medicate away the relentless anger and frustration. He cursed himself for the weight he'd put on, for wasting his time and money on therapy, for being a 'worthless piece of shit'.

He drew figures within geometric shapes, trying to calm himself, then mocked his 'shit drawings'. His moods swung. He later said he felt guilty for letting me down.

The next week, I sat waiting for him in my room as the clock showed five then ten past the hour. Afternoon sunshine began to slip through the window and across the desk and I thought I might not be seeing

William again. I read back over pages in my notebook looking for clues, things I might have said, things I might have overlooked. His words, the routines and rituals of meetings were but part of the story, so to speak. Being late, being early, missing sessions, withholding payments, or over-paying, these were all part of the process, part of an attempt to try to understand and change long-ingrained and unhelpful patterns.

Tutting when I couldn't read what I'd written, I shut my eyes and dropped the useless notebook in my lap.

———•———

Meanwhile William argued with himself, go, don't go. He couldn't find any peace. To get away he drove up the high-sided narrow Chiltern roads, lanes once cut into the hills by horse-drawn carts. He drove up through Turville and along Christmas Common. There he walked in the woods trying to find answers to his problems amongst the bluebells. Back in his car his sneering face gazed back at him from the mirror, it hissed 'Why don't you just top yourself you useless cunt?'

He drove back through High Wycombe. By the hospital at the round-about, while he queued to make his way home, a group of uniformed girls crossed in front of him. They were walking to the grammar school and he saw that behind them, one girl walked by herself, she stayed near to the flint wall, head down, closed off, trying to make herself invisible. He later said that he saw his shame and isolation in her, that it was seeing her that made him think twice about throwing the towel in, and he decided not to go home, instead, he drove his conflicting thoughts and feelings to my room. He arrived twenty minutes late. As soon as he came in he started telling me stories, it was like he'd come to confession.

———•———

'When I was small, my friend Neil and I were chased by some boys, we ran to his house, but before we got there his father appeared at the back door. I thought his dad was angry with us, but he was angry with the boys that'd scared us.'

I could see he was still surprised about it now and I wondered if William thought I was going to tell him off for missing last week's session.

'Neil told his dad what had happened and his dad ran to find them. I'd never seen anyone run as fast, like a man possessed, arms and legs pumping, I found it frightening. He caught two of them and dragged them back across the field. I remember feeling uncomfortable and thinking this is wrong, you shouldn't treat me like this. I don't deserve it.'

'He thought you did,' I said.

'He was called Stan, he was the sort of man my father would have looked down on. I didn't tell my parents about it, I never took problems home. I spent a lot of time trying to be helpful at home. I had another friend, we used to draw together, his father drew cartoons for a newspaper. My friend Paul got out this big roll of paper and pushed it across his bedroom floor, it rolled all the way to the door. He said, "Come on, let's draw, we can draw what we want." I was excited but I had this overpowering sense that I shouldn't. I've always felt that around creative things. I sometimes get an impulse to draw or make something and almost immediately this feeling that I'm not allowed to comes over me. His father liked me, he drew me a birthday card, a cartoon version of me standing on a snooker table hitting the balls with a golf club.'

'Sounds like he knew something about your feelings for golf clubs,' I said. William smiled.

'I didn't show it to my father. I'm aware of these memories coming back to me. It's good remembering these things, but why can't I keep hold of them when I leave?' The question hung between us, interrupted from outside by a screech of cars breaking, a long blast from a car horn rang out, then a shout, then another, angry men, road rage.

'I have this image of a mallet smashing up my ideas,' said William. 'Any sign of an impulse to do something and this massive über mallet comes crashing down. I can work, I can do things for other people, but nothing for me.'

'It's something that it let you come back here,' I said.

'It can be different here,' said William, 'but when I leave it gets me, and then the only thing I can do is drink, attack myself with drink. I don't even like drinking that much. I was thinking about making a kind of trompe l'oeil image, thought I'd give myself the target of sending it to the Royal Academy Summer Exhibition, but the über mallet got me. I ended up hiding all the art materials, then I drank. I carried on doing things around the house, making supper, making sure everything was nice for Meg, I sat watching television programmes I have no interest in when I could be working on ideas.'

'You can do things for others, but apart from that you're alone with destructive drinking rituals.'

'Alone with my destructive rituals,' William repeated. He nodded to himself, 'I thought I should just send the Royal Academy an enormous wooden mallet. Exhibit A, My Über Mallet. I could send them a bottle of gin to go with it.' I thought that sounded apt. William looked at the floor, quiet for a few moments. 'I'm sorry about not coming last week. I just couldn't come. I ignored your email, I should've got back to you.'

'That's ok,' I said, 'you can't say much to an über mallet.' William gave me a half smile. I was aware that there must have been a break in the cloud because the afternoon sun moved across the window and I noticed William watching a gold rectangle that spread across the couch.

'Does anybody use that couch?'

'What do you think?'

William grunted.

'What do I think? Maybe. I wouldn't. I wasn't sure about coming here when I saw that.'

'You should have said.'

William smiled.

'If my twin was here, I could imagine saying to him "use the couch, rest, recover." Other people can have things like that, not me.'

'You said everything went wrong at school, but these memories are older than that.'

William remained fixed on the rectangle of light on the couch.

'These rituals,' I continued, 'the drinking, the über mallet, I think these are older than school too.' He shifted forward in his chair.

'At primary school someone's duffel bag hit me in the stomach, I'd never been winded before, I couldn't breathe, I thought I was dying. But I remember thinking that I shouldn't ask for help, that it would be better if I took myself off and died on my own, that if I asked for help something worse might happen.' He spread his hands in front of him, mouth open. 'I was only about six.' He swallowed, put his hands on the arms of the chair and looked out of the window. 'If that happened to someone else, another boy, if it happened to you, I'd say "Shit, are you alright? What's happened? Let's get help." I'd want to help. Yet if I ask for help for me, something worse might happen. What's that about?'

I noticed I'd become a friend of William's in the story.

'I didn't deserve help. I still don't, I'm outside the rest of humanity. What I'd like is for a surgeon to snip the hot-wire that runs through my brain, I've always thought that must be how ECT works. People who've had shock treatment talk about their memories being disrupted, that they lose some of their depression because they no longer remember what depressed them.' He turned to look back at the light on the couch. 'That makes a lot of sense to me. I wish I could hang onto the things that interest me, but I know when I leave that I won't.' William turned back to the light gliding across the couch. A bird landed on the roof, I tracked its movements. 'I couldn't face you last week. But I have arranged to speak with a photographer, someone local. He seemed to understand what I was talking about. The perspective image, the trompe l'oeil effect. I've been meaning to follow up on that for ages. I may need to move our session, if I keep coming. It depends when he can fit me in.'

'Right, I said, feeling my heart sink. I might have become his friend, but I didn't understand him. 'We can see what we can do.'

'I've got an idea about making advertising posters, optical illusions that draw the viewer in. I don't want to say too much. Don't want to jinx it. It felt good to organise it.'

'Yes, I can see.'

'It might be a good outcome for these sessions, getting into a creative project. This has been ok, talking here, I wouldn't have looked up the photographer without having spoken here. But I think this might be making things worse.'

'Right,' I said. I heard a noise above and saw a magpie fly away, I remember thinking 'one for sorrow,' I sensed the tide of the conversation running away from us.

'Talking here, sometimes I get interested, sometimes I remember things, feelings, but when I leave everything resets.' William looked out of the window and then back at me. 'No, it's stronger than that, it's more than a reset, it's violent. In the car, I flip into nasty critical thoughts, then I drive home and drink gin in secret. That's got worse since I've been seeing you.'

'I think two things are happening,' I said, 'in one you remember and make connections, in the other you attack yourself, a bit like in the Stan story. It's like you accidentally make a valuable connection with yourself, but then you react because you feel you don't deserve it. Or with Paul, you feel you don't deserve to draw what you want. I wondered if that is what's going on with the photography.'

'You think I shouldn't do it?'

'It sounds like something you want to do, but it made me think of you needing to find someone who understands you better than I do. It sounds like it might stop you coming here.'

'And you don't think I should do that?' William asked. 'Shouldn't stop coming here?'

'No,' I said. 'I don't.'

'Oh,' said William, pulling a mock face, 'an opinion.' His eyes skimmed over the knots in the walls. 'I can't come here forever.'

'I don't think you'll come here forever, but I think you've got more engaged in working here than you thought you would, and at the moment that seems to coincide with a pressure to attack yourself.'

'Stopping this would be attacking myself?'

'I think that's involved. Not the whole story, as I say I can see you want to work on your photography.' William gave a sigh.

'I don't know,' he spread his fingers out. 'I might ring him, see if he could meet another day.' He leant back in his chair, shut his eyes. 'I hadn't thought that I was putting myself in my place, not with the photography, but it might have led to me breaking off here, it's strange the way you come at things.' He glanced at the Van Gogh print. 'Is it time to stop? It must be about time.'

'Almost,' I said, regretting the fact.

William gathered up his things and left me looking at the empty chair. *An opinion.* Then I checked my watch, reached for my pen and drew a picture of a stickman in a wood smashing up a shed with an oversized über mallet.

But the thing that most interested me was that he'd missed a session and then come back. He'd decided to stop and then changed his mind, that was unusual. Plenty of people stop psychotherapy prematurely, maybe most people, but not many come back. I felt that this suggested that William might have become more engaged than he realised; clearly things were still in the balance, but coming back was unusual. Still, there were the critical aggressive destructive feelings, the über mallet, but there was more than that: I felt we were onto something, developing elements of trust.

William remained attached to the idea that there was something wrong with him, whereas I thought that things had happened to him. I tried not to rush him, to a significant degree it was beyond my control, but him coming back made me think that a defence had softened, and that there might be more for him here.

In therapy, problems sometimes need to be worked on until a more benign position is developed. Evidence of such benign development is the establishment of trust, and the wish, the emergent capacity, to reveal more. It takes care to nurture and create such benign therapeutic moments and getting past the über mallet and deciding to come back was such a moment.

I was aware how interested I'd become in our work. I discussed it in supervision, I had presented it at various case discussions, and I could see that other people were interested too.

Chapter 4

'These sessions might be having an effect on me,' said William. 'Meg and I went for a curry. Three men at a table near us started telling misogynistic jokes. I got annoyed, stared at them. The one who was telling the jokes couldn't see me, but his friend did, he stared back and for a moment I thought we might be on the verge of a confrontation, but I wasn't backing down. Then he dropped his gaze, turned to his friend, and quietened him down. I was surprised, then I relaxed, drank some lagers, but I didn't drink in secret when we got home. When we walked back up the road Meg said how relaxed I was, she said me coming here has made a difference, she didn't see what happened, but I did feel good. It's unlike me to express anger.' William put his glasses, keys, and wallet on the table beside him, the light in the room dimmed, clouds gathering. 'Well of course I do, but only towards myself. The über mallet, the secret drinking, that goes on. But that night, when we walked back up the high street, I felt good, different. It's unusual that I'd feel like that. Do you see what I'm saying?'

'This was different,' I said.

'Exactly. And I don't think it would have happened if I wasn't coming here. There was something about the feeling, it was … appropriate.'

'Appropriate.' I echoed the word back to him. William leant forward, elbows on his knees.

'I can't tell you how unusual it is for me to feel like that.' He smiled, I smiled back. 'I never have appropriate feelings about myself,' said William.

'It sounds like the way you've spoken about being complimented,' I said.

'Yep, no compliments or appropriate feelings. Why? I've always thought that it was because I'm bad in some way, that there is something wrong with me.'

'I don't think it's because there's something wrong with you, but I do think things may have happened to you.'

'It's not that there's something wrong with me. It's that something has happened to me,' repeated William, 'that's what you mean?'

'Yes. You're so caught up thinking there is something wrong with you that you're never free to say more about what's happened to you.'

A frown moved across William's brow.

'You think that things have happened to me, which I think are my fault?'

'It wasn't your fault that the men were telling misogynistic jokes.'

'Normally I shouldn't be angry, I shouldn't glare at them, but this was different.'

'It sounds like it may have been appropriate.'

'You're saying it's like the other thing, it's not that there is something wrong with me?' said William.

'Yes.'

'That things have happened to me.' William repeated it to himself. He scratched his head, his phone fell from his pocket and onto the floor, he picked it up and put it on the table. 'Normally I'd apologise for dropping that, but I won't.' He let out a tiny, muted sob, bent forward and covered his face with his hand. 'I'm welling up,' he sniffed, 'I want to shut the feelings down, it's like being given a compliment, like I'm feeling something I shouldn't. I want to shut it down.'

'I'm not sure that you should.' It was the first time he'd cried in one of our sessions.

William wiped his eyes with a tissue, lowered his hand, rocked back in his chair and went back to looking out of the window. 'This time is fine by the way, let's keep this time. If that's ok with you?'

'Right,' I said.

'In fact, I wondered if you ever see people more than once a week. I think it might help if I came more often. Just to see what it's like. If you could? Might speed things up.'

'Let's have a look.' I reached for my diary. 'In a way,' I said, 'it seems like you've been shown something now, the feeling that welled up. I think it fits with feeling annoyed at the restaurant too.'

William mulled that over. 'Do you think it's linked with wanting to come here more often?'

'It might be, you're coming here, you're trying to set up the meeting with the photographer, you're trying to …'

'This sounds a bit close to a compliment, compliments aren't for me,' said William, staring at me. I thought of the men in the restaurant.

'I can compliment you,' said William, 'but I don't want to be complimented.'

'No.' I turned his logic over in my mind.

'You've said something interesting though,' agreed William.

'Is this you complimenting me?' I asked. William smiled.

'Yes, that's how it works, I can compliment you, and I am, because you've said something interesting; it's not that there are things wrong with me; it's that things have happened to me.' He sat back in his chair, glanced at the Van Gogh. I wished I'd never put the picture up.

William looked at his watch, then the window. He turned back to me.

'I saw the photographer, then later I worked on my project. The maths is complex, getting the numbers right, and when I thought I had it, I printed a test. You have to fold the image carefully, and I was looking at the print, looking at where to fold it, suddenly I had this strong feeling that I was in trouble, my heart was racing,' he looked up at me, 'but in fact, I'd done something right. It was a success, the image I mean. And it was the success that was wrong, that's where the trouble was. The next moment I shut it all in a drawer, emailed the photographer and said I wouldn't be going back. I drank a lot, all weekend, drank in secret too.' William shut his eyes and put his head back. I wondered how often I'd been close to getting an email like that.

'I'm sorry to hear that,' I said.

He reached into his pocket and took out a piece of paper and held it out to me. 'I drew this.' I looked at the image, I saw a triangle, I couldn't make out the details. 'It's a boy folded in on himself, in a triangle.

A worthless triangle boy. Me.' William put the image back in his pocket and turned back to the pine walls.

'I have this memory, when I was small, I'm with my mother, and she's being cuddly. I don't like thinking about it. I start to think about being with her, then it's gone. I don't know. I spoke to my elder sister, she said I was with my mother when she became ill.'

'Do you know what she is referring to?'

'My sister said she thought my mother had a miscarriage, that I was with her when it happened.' William laced his fingers together, a silence developed, he made a shallow cough. 'Dad swore us to secrecy. You asked me about the gap between me and my younger sister, I suppose it was a big gap.'

'Eight years I think you said.'

'Do you think that means something? I've wondered whether my father was violent to her. He had a temper, he was very physical with us, he liked to put us in our place.'

'That's what you say when you speak about flipping, you put yourself in your place.'

'If I think you're complimenting me, I react. It shouldn't be happening to me. Not my place.'

'Your triangle place?' I said.

———•———

Being able to draw and show me the picture of himself in the triangle marked a turning point in our work together; it was another benign therapeutic moment. It wasn't just that he was revealing something, it was that he did so via a picture; I knew that typically there were severe prohibitions, über mallets, blocking his creativity.

Now we'd established a new level of trust, and from here, and based on the information he was able to check with his brother and sister, we were able to piece together his early childhood in greater detail.

This was the first time William spoke about these things. They were important, particularly in the context of his adult emotional experience: the persistent low mood that had brought him to me in the first place.

Part II

William's early life

Chapter 5

Leicester, July 1966

It's late on a Sunday afternoon and the Smith family are together in their sitting room in Leicester.

Sunshine from two west-facing windows slants across the floor. William's mother is translating a passage from a Greek textbook at her table, his father is reading the paper. His brother, Graham, has stopped trying to build a house out of the coloured blocks and has joined his sister. They are trying to put an oversized wooden jigsaw of a farm together. They argue over some of the pieces, then slot them together; now there are two pink pigs and the beginnings of a fence.

Across from them, William toddles, moving from chair to chair. He is concentrating, mumbling to himself and a large cuddly grey black dog that hangs from his mouth by a saliva-soaked ear. William makes noises as he moves and calls out indistinct half words. He opens his mouth and the dog falls. He lets go of his chair and shifts to face his mother. He takes a step towards her, then another, then falls flat on his face into the sunlight, like he is falling into a paddling pool. He shrieks with laughter, his brother and sister laugh.

'William's funny!' says his sister, Flo.

'Look at William, he's funny mummy!' says Graham, then to his sister, 'look Flo there's another stinky pig.'

'William's doggy stinks,' says Flo, screwing up her nose. She looks at the piece Graham's pointing at and makes a grunting sound.

His mother makes a distracted noise but doesn't look up. His father mumbles something from behind his paper and starts to fold the page to get at the crossword; he stretches his arm, flexes his hand. It is unusual that his father is present; but for an elbow strain he'd be at the golf club.

William stands, he squints, he raises a hand to shield his eyes from the sunlight, and sways back towards the chair. He rests for a moment, his weight balanced loose against it. With each movement of his chubby legs and body he emits sounds, half-formed words, an enthusiastic commentary on the afternoon. He is happy, he toddles, falls and laughs again. This time his mother turns to look at him and smiles, she looks across at her husband who is absorbed in the crossword. William shouts louder and more high-pitched. Graham laughs, Flo tries to mimic the high-pitched noise.

William starts to repeat the process once more.

His mother turns back to her books but as she does so, she doubles over on herself in a sudden movement. She cries out and tries to swallow the sound back with one hand covering her mouth, the other tight against her stomach. The noise is strange and sharp. Everyone stops what they are doing and looks at her; even William's father, who hates fuss, lowers his paper to see what's happened.

William hears her cry out and, balancing as he is, turns to look. He sees her bent over, leaning forwards across her chair. He starts to toddle towards her, making noises as he does so, he's not sure what's happened but he wants to join in, he wants to play, he wants more laughter. He falls over, arms spread, shrieking, at the very same moment that his mother falls out of her chair and onto the floor next to him. They are nearly nose to nose. William is almost hysterical with laughter, he loves it when he can get her to join in with his games.

In an instant, William's father reaches down, scoops him around the middle, and the next thing he knows he is being rushed out of the room and up to his bedroom. It's like the flying game but it's less fun, he can hardly breathe. His father is moving fast and is rough with him.

William bounces against his hip as they rush into the hallway and climb the stairs to the landing. They reach William's bedroom in seconds, where he is dropped, not onto his new bed, but into his old faded buttermilk yellow cot. Dazed by the speed of events, William just manages to turn and call out 'Daddy!' as the door shuts on him. He hears his father pace back towards the landing.

William hauls himself up against the bars of his cot and stands, confused, shaking. He calls out to the empty room, the firmly closed door, his family beyond.

There is no reply.

He cries and then wets himself, it soaks through his nappy, through his blue shorts and runs down his legs. He calls out again. And again. He lurches around on the mattress and shouts. He doesn't like being in his cot, he sleeps in the bed now.

He waits, he gets no reply, he slumps down.

William doesn't want the door shut, he's too lonely. He doesn't know why his father has done that. It's one thing being in his room with the door open, but quite another when it's shut, he feels cut off. He calls out again, he shouts anything he can think of, he wants his father to come back and take him downstairs, he wants them all to be together again laughing, he wants to make them all laugh. Then he remembers doggy, his comforter.

'Doggy's downstairs! doggy's downstairs!' he shouts, then quieter, to himself, 'I miss doggy.' He puts both hands on the bars of the cot and calls out, 'Mummy!' then he calls 'Daddy!' then 'Doggy!' He shouts their names over and over.

There is no reply. No one comes. He sucks his thumb.

He plays the waiting game, where he waits and is patient and then when he is a good boy he gets the good thing, like the mashed-up eggs on soldiers when they're ready, not when he wants them. He plays the waiting game for a long time, he's never played it for so long, he doesn't think anybody has. He tries to be quiet, patient, to be a good boy, but he can feel all of the fun of the afternoon slipping away from him. His nappy and shorts are wet and uncomfortable and his bottom is cold and sore. His mother hasn't put the cream on him.

The afternoon light starts to turn now, the yellow fades, weaker than it was downstairs.

He thinks it can't be bedtime because he hasn't had his bath yet, and for a moment the thought gives him hope, but it doesn't last. His head hangs forward, heavy, pressed against the bars. He slumps down on the mattress. In time, he falls asleep, curled up, sucking his thumb.

———————•———————

Sometime later he is woken by a sound from somewhere in the house. A door slam? Was it his door? Were they with him in his room? Are they outside his room? His mouth is dry and sticky, he says 'Mummy.' There is no reply. He climbs up, leans against the bars and calls out again. He calls 'Mummy, Mummy' until his words start to get mixed up. 'Mummy, Murry, Mummy, Murry, Mummy, Murry, Mummy, Murry.' He calls out, over and over, falling into a rhythm. The longer he says it, the more unhappy it sounds. He doesn't know what he is saying anymore. If they come he won't be cross, he will make them laugh and laugh, he will make everything better, he will pull himself up and toddle and fall, they love that. He will make them all happy and doggy will be happy too. He shouts, 'I want doggy.'

But still they don't come. He plays the waiting game again but his heart isn't in it.

It is darker now but the curtains are still open. He doesn't understand it, they always shut the curtains, there are elephants on them and he always says goodnight to the elephants, and good morning too, but now there's just the dark window. William is unhappy about the elephants.

'I'm sad mummy,' he says to the empty room.

He can't make sense of it. He can't make sense of the elephants. Try as he can, he can only see the edges of their trunks and ears, he wishes he had doggy, they could look together. He likes it when the elephants look at him and doggy. He starts to think that maybe the elephants don't like him, that they have turned their backs on him. He doesn't know why they would do that. He sits alone with his questions.

Has he done something bad? Has he got everything wrong? Are the elephants and his family cross with him? Maybe they didn't like him falling over and toddling around the sitting room and shouting? Is doggy cross with him? He doesn't like these thoughts at all.

He sits up and rocks forward, stretches his fingers out, but it's no good. Once he's thought it, it keeps coming back; are they cross with him? He looks around his cot, rocks his head from side to side. He looks at the door, he pleads with it to open. Then a new thought, worse still, occurs to him: 'Did I make mummy angry?', 'Did she fall out of her chair because she was angry with me?'

The thoughts gang up on him. He's thirsty, he wants water, milk, he wants everything to be different. He feels sick and scared. He wants the thoughts to go away.

He shouts out the joking noises that they like. He won't stop shouting until they come, or he falls asleep.

———•———

A bad dream wakes him. In the dream the elephants closed his curtains and told him to shut up, they were rough with him, they put the blanket right over his head. He tried to stand up and reach out, then he fell. It was a scary dream, like the one he had about the clowns.

He sits up, now more awake, then he sees that his curtains have been shut, and it all comes back to him. He thinks Mummy or Daddy must have come when he was asleep. He starts to cry again, he wants to see Mummy, wants to hide under the blankets with Mummy, wants to get away from the silence.

'Go boo Mummy,' he says. 'Mummy likes that. Go boo. I'm tired Mummy.' He wants Mummy to come and make everything better, he searches in vain for something to make it better.

He is cold and hungry. It is dark and there is a thin strip of orange light across the ceiling, it reaches into the corner of the room. He knows that is the streetlight. He's puzzled. He shouts out.

'Stweet light.' He points, he shouts 'stweet light!' He thought it was odd because the elephant curtains should have stopped it. Then he remembers, and things don't feel funny, and he has the tummy pain, and he is sore and he feels panicky again. He calls 'Mummy Murry, Mummy Murry, Mummy Murry, Mummy Murry,' he tries to settle himself but can't. He bangs his head against the bars, it hurts but it makes a loud knocking noise. He thinks they must hear that. Now they'll rescue me. He thinks, 'I'll bang my head and they'll come and Mummy, and everything will be better again.' He mumbles 'Mummy, Murry, Mummy, Murry, Mummy, Murry.' His head goes 'knock! knock! knock!' on the bars.

———•———

William tapped his hand on the arm of the chair, then seemed to become aware of the noise he was making and stopped.

'I don't know what I'm telling you, I'm not sure what happened,' he bowed his head.

'I think I see that,' I said. 'I think it's hard to know quite what you went through.'

'It wouldn't stop, I couldn't make it stop.'

From somewhere outside, the cry of a red kite stretched out alone and friendless in the air.

William's head leant against his hand, his fingertips rubbed at a point on his forehead.

'I think that's remained the problem, I don't think it has stopped,' I said.

'I think I sort of lost myself, it makes me feel sick just to think about it. Why didn't they come?' He closed his eyes. I tried to picture the bedroom, William distressed, waiting in the dark. William tapped on the arm of the chair, I felt myself drawn back to the knocking sound deep in the house.

Blank-faced, William looked across at me, raised his shoulders, then let them drop back down, dejected.

'Everything changed,' said William, 'I couldn't seem to fit in. I felt I had to be in my place, keep everything to myself. I think it's still going on now, when I have time on my hands, that's when it gets me. It's like a force inside me, a sort of squashed uncomfortable feeling.'

'It makes me think of something traumatic and claustrophobic,' I said. 'That you were stuck in this and that's how it remained, with no apparent way out.'

'Other people could have things, I couldn't, I couldn't even have my cuddly dog, my parents threw it out, they said it stank. It's as if I was thrown away, who I was, the me I was before.' William sat up, and turned his chair away from me, he closed his eyes and sighed.

'Do you know what happened to your mother?' I asked. 'You said you remember her falling, do you know what happened?' William shook his head.

'No. I haven't thought about any of this in a long time. I don't think it's ever been discussed, not with me. I told you my sister once said some-thing, I think she remembered it. My brother once started talking to me at a family wedding, years after it all happened. He got quite emotional, he'd been drinking. He went to live in New York to get away from my dad. It was curious, coincidental, because we both flew to the wedding from the USA, different flights, I was on the West Coast. He started talking about how he'd tried to get Mum's attention. He got upset, said he remembered how he tried to get her to go up to me. But we weren't a family that talked about things. Or we weren't after then.' He raised his eyes, spread his hands. 'I don't know, something happened and everything changed and after that home wasn't the same. I wasn't me anymore, I was just an imitation me, doing everything for everybody else.' He opened his mouth, paused, then said, 'I don't know if there is any point going over all this.'

I felt the weight of defeat. I wondered about what had happened to William's mother but I wasn't sure if there was any point trying to ask more.

'There wasn't anything you could do to change it back then,' I said.

'Talking here sometimes does something for me,' said William. 'If I remember something, tell you about it, it has an effect. An energy, I don't know, something like that, but when I leave, I revert, I attack myself. After I showed you the triangle picture I got in my car, and as soon as I looked in the mirror I became consumed by shame, self-hatred, anger.' He broke off and looked at the knots in the walls.

I learnt later that he would sometimes see faces and shapes in the knots in the wooden panelling. He saw one of them start to contort and resemble Munch's *The Scream*. William swivelled his chair back to face me. 'And I'm drinking way too much. I think my wife is worried about my drinking.' He looked at the floor, silent. I looked at his thinning hair, I was aware of how unhappy the situation was.

'Things are very bad at the moment,' I said.

'Not at the moment,' said William, looking up, an edge in his voice, 'always. Always.' He paused, clenched his jaw. 'I don't think you get that.' He stared hard at me.

'This is going on all the time,' I said. William turned to look back out of the window. 'I think, like you say, there are moments when it changes, like when you wrote the legal letter, or sometimes here, in the session, the mood will change.'

'But it never lasts,' William came back at me. 'And when it returns it's worse. It might change for a moment, but it doesn't stop.'

'I think that's what it was like in the early memories you describe, unexpected moments in which things are suddenly alright, good even. But they don't last.'

'That's what makes it worse,' said William.

'And it's like what's happening here. Out of the blue your mood might lift here, the energy like you say, but then when you leave something will put you back in your place.'

'I'm not meant to have this,' said William. I could see that. I wondered if he might be about to get up and leave, I knew we were at a delicate point. 'Good things are for other people,' said William. He turned his chair until he was facing the couch, he pointed. 'If my imaginary twin had gone through all this and was here sitting on your couch telling us about it, I'd feel sorry for him. I'd say, "oh no, poor you." But I can't have this,' he jabbed at his chest. 'I can't have good things. And what I worry about is that talking here just makes everything worse. I come here, I talk, then I leave, I revert.' William gave a half laugh. 'Sometimes I think I am coming here for you, not me, that I'm just coming to tell you these things. Like I am trying to make things better for you, make you feel like you do a good job.' William paused. 'When I leave I feel worse. Is there any point to this? Tell me what the point of this is? Going over it all? Am I suddenly going to feel better about everything?' He lent forward, his chair rocked under his weight, I thought he might topple over. 'You don't know what to say to that do you?' said William.

'Well,' I said, trying to pick my words with care.

William tapped the arm of the chair, interrupting, 'I feel pretty fed up with this.'

'I can see that.'

William raised his voice.

'Is this a plan to try to make me angry with you? Is that how this works? I get angry with you?'

'I don't think I'd call it a plan,' I said, 'but I think you had to take your anger out on yourself, and you still do, when you leave here, the flip. I think anger is part of what keeps you in your place.' William stared at me. 'I wonder if that is part of where the über mallet came from?'

I could see William thinking the idea over.

'I think, as it were,' I said, 'that some kind of system developed that works to keep you in your place. There's a dominant idea that you should be good, as though if you'd been good, you wouldn't have been left in the cot. I think it developed out of the experiences you've described. An idea that if you don't stay in your place something bad will happen. Something will get out of hand. And that something like that could happen here.'

'That I shouldn't be telling you these things?' said William.

'I don't think they are things that anyone listened to when you were young. And back then you would have done everything to try to keep your mother and father happy. Back then you had to stick to the story, your rituals.'

'I am not keeping to rituals here,' said William, 'that's for sure. Bringing the triangle boy picture. When I tell you about things, the memories, the bits and pieces, I start linking things together. I couldn't do that back then. When I've told you, then I feel conflicted. Part of me wants to leave, but part of me wants to keep on talking with you. But really whatever I do, when I leave and get in my car, I'll flip, I'll take it out on myself. I'll buy more booze, drink more. And tomorrow morning when I look in the mirror I'll be cursing myself again. That triangle drawing is me, the boy folded up on himself, that's me. Every time that bedroom door shut on me I was more convinced that I wasn't good enough.' William stared at me, then he lowered his gaze and looked away, his fingers tapped on the arm of the chair.

Chapter 6

Flo's wedding, 1985

William sat alone near the back of the room. He undid his top button and took off his tie, he was drinking sparkling water and regretting he'd given up smoking. His brother Graham slumped into the chair next to him just managing to balance a glass of brandy which he held out to William. William raised his glass in return, they clinked. Graham set his glass down and ran a hand through his hair. 'Dancing Queen' started to play and a man on the other side of the room threw his arms in the air and joined the dancers on the floor, the lights changed in time to the music, and a spinning mirror ball sent tiny coloured discs off orbiting the room. Their parents sat with a group at one of the tables across from them.

'When are you back to the States?'

'I'm not,' said William, slipping his tie into his jacket pocket, 'I'm not sure what I'm doing next.'

'Brave man. I'm back to New York next week. I always feel better having the Atlantic between me and Dad.' A bit late to the joke, William smiled, half laughed; the years apart had left an awkward distance between them. 'I'm glad you came William, I wanted to speak to you.' Graham turned in his chair and in an uncommonly intimate gesture put his left hand on William's right hand, he gave it a brief squeeze and then let go. William, surprised by the touch, momentarily turned to look at Graham and then back to watch the lights spinning across the walls.

'I wanted to say sorry William.'

William looked at him, he wasn't sure where Graham was going, he wondered if this was the drink talking.

'Thing is, I wasn't a good enough brother to you. All that stuff that went on at home. I try to put it out of my mind, but I think it's part of why I drink so much. Do you think about it?' William half considered the question: he didn't tend to think about the past, if he did it just reminded him of how bad he felt about himself. Graham drank some brandy and put the glass down on the table.

'The nearer the wedding got it all started to come back to me again, the way you were left in your room, ignored. I did try to get mum to go to you, but she was always in her books, all that ancient Greek. I'd hear you making those noises, knocking, I hated the noise, and I'd tell her but she wouldn't listen. She knew more about Thucydides than us.' William smiled, sipped his water, he wasn't sure if he wanted to get into this conversation, he watched the lights. He looked at the bubbles in his glass then at Flo on the dance floor, she looked happy. He felt Graham lean into him.

'I started having nightmares, like something from an Edgar Allen Poe story, always set in our old home, outside Leicester. Someone being locked in a room. I knew they were about you and me, I hated that house. I ended up in therapy in New York, spent a fortune with some man who never said anything. I managed to find someone more human in the end.'

Despite the music and the spinning lights, William listened.

'And the thing is, I remember going up to you and finding your door shut, and I tried to get Mum to come but she never helped. Do you remember all that? I hope you don't mind me telling you this, I thought it might help me if I told you about it. I thought if I told you then the dreams might stop.'

William wasn't sure what to say to him, he knew he should say something.

'Nasty dreams Graham.' He looked back at the lights circling the room. The lights had a calming effect on him, he turned back to Graham.

'I don't know, I don't remember much from back then, I tried to put it out of my mind.'

Later, William said goodnight to Graham and left the wedding party. Then he went up to his room and drank everything in the minibar.

———•———

'Maybe all of my rituals started in that cot,' said William, shifting in his chair. 'All the head-banging, name-saying, all that Mummy Murry stuff. Lying under the blankets, rocking my head from side to side saying made up words, my own Greek words, maybe the über mallet too.'

'That might be right,' I said, 'I think these are very old rituals.'

'I remember when I saw a film of the Romanian orphans, the children in their cots. I could see their distress, I mean I think everyone could, but I felt I knew it too. I sort of related to them, banging their heads, I could see they were traumatised. When I saw those images I felt shame, I felt very uncomfortable about it.' He turned his hands into fists and then stretched his fingers out, he rubbed the palms of his hands together, they made a sibilant seashore noise.

'I can see the distress for other people,' said William, still chafing his palms, 'but I can't see it relates to me.'

'You don't think about yourself having gone through trauma.'

'No, I can see other people might have. If it was anyone else I would see it, but not me.' William leant back in his chair, he swivelled it slowly from side to side.

It began to rain, soft at first. I thought there was some comfort in the sound, the pair of us sitting together listening to the rain. Glancing at William as I did so, I turned my head to watch the small leaves of the olive tree dance when the rain drops fell on them. The olive tree made me think of William's mother reading Greek to herself, away in her hobby, of William left alone. William listened to the rain too.

'When I was still at the little school,' said William, 'with my brother and sister, one day we walked home in the rain, we got soaked. My brother was walking a bit ahead, my sister was holding my hand, I was worried about what was going to happen when we got home. We came across the gravel, up to the house, and my mother was standing, waiting, I thought she would be angry about how wet we were, but she couldn't have been more pleased to see us. All of us. And she was saying,

"Come on, upstairs, quick." I thought I was going to be put in my room, but I wasn't, she had run a bath, a big deep hot bath. She helped us get out of our wet clothes and we all got in. I couldn't believe it.'

I could hear his surprise.

'We were all happy, and my mother was happy. And it got better. She got us out of the bath, wrapped us up in towels, and then we put our pyjamas on and went downstairs and she made us boiled eggs and toast. I loved that, and we were all sitting around the kitchen table all happy and warm, and she was happy. And I thought "Thank goodness, it's all over." But it wasn't.' He watched the rain falling outside, it was heavier now, audible on the roof. 'I haven't thought of that in a long time. Why couldn't it stay like that? I don't remember what happened the rest of that day. I don't know what made her do that. It didn't last. I was soon back in my room again, I don't think I could understand what had happened to my mother, we weren't joined up anymore. I know she used to like being soppy, and I remember that rainy day. Why couldn't she be more like that?'

I could see William had never been able to predict her moods: one moment loving, the next withdrawn, isolating, away in her books. Love then no love. He never knew how she kept him in mind. Not quite the good enough mother. A woman who needed help herself.

'I think that made it all the more confusing, tantalising, never know-ing what you would get from your mother,' I said.

'The only answer I could find was that it was my fault. That I must have done something, so I kept trying to do things to make every-thing better. Like I used to tidy up after meals, my brother and sister didn't do that, they didn't think they were bad or that it was their job to tidy everything up. I was smaller than them but after meals I would clean up, I tried to make everything right. If everything could just be fine, just like it was that day. I was always doing things that I thought would help.'

He trailed off and glanced at the clock. I could see there were ten minutes left. I watched William working through his thoughts. I thought over the details of the story, I wondered if we might sit in silence till the end. I had an incomplete idea about William and the traumas he described. I felt I should say something, but couldn't get the thought straight in my mind; weighing the balance up, I decided not to speak.

In the quiet my gaze drifted above William's shoulder and out of the window behind him. I could just see the bird box on the hornbeam, I wondered if any birds were sheltering there. I could see the beginnings of autumn. I thought of all the leaves I would soon have to clear up, all the work to try to keep everything tidy; it was always me that had to clear the leaves up. I heard William pick up the theme.

'I was always trying to make everything right. When we got pocket money on Saturday morning we would go to the shops, my brother and sister would buy sweets for themselves. Not me. I used to find things, gifts to buy for my mother and father, it didn't cross my mind that I could buy something for me, a comic, sweets. All the effort I was going to, to make everything nice for them. If someone else was telling me these stories I would feel sorry for them. I'd think it awful, some poor child desperate to make everything better.' I thought of the burden William was carrying, trying to look after his family's needs. 'Other people's homes weren't like mine, other children at school didn't have to do everything for their families. At primary school the headmaster said that we could bring packed lunches and I rushed home to tell my mother, I was so pleased, the food was so awful, but she was cross when I told her. Said I would have to make them myself. I was embarrassed. And the next day I got up early and made my own sandwiches. We used to keep the butter in the fridge, a big hard block of it. I tried to make Marmite sandwiches and the bread tore as I spread the butter. My friends had these immaculate lunch boxes, I had an Action Man lunch box. I remember how worried I was that I would drop it, and everyone would see. They all had their neatly wrapped sandwiches, an apple, snacks. I could see the effort that their mothers had gone to, they were showing off how good they were, how good their children were. I sat on my own and ate my shit sandwiches, that's what they looked like, shit. All torn bread and messy and wrapped up in that horrible grease-proof paper we used to have, it was like the toilet paper we had at school. Shit sandwiches wrapped in toilet paper. I couldn't understand my mother. She'd changed, I'd changed, everything had changed.'

'Yes, I can see that it had, and fixing it was beyond your control.'

'Everything was different, we were changed,' said William.

'Something valuable had been lost from your home,' I said.

'Vulnerable?' said William.

'I said valuable, but I think you were vulnerable too.'

'I can't think like that about myself. When I did things for them I felt closer to the rest of humanity. I didn't get pleasure from it but it made me feel safer. Nothing would go right. I remember my dad coming to my primary school, looking around my classroom. I was excited to have him there, to show him my letters. We were learning handwriting. I'd put a lot of work into it. And I showed him, I got him to sit down at the table on the little chair. "Dad look, look how neat my letters are, look at them." I was proud that I'd managed to do the letters right. I loved the way they flowed, that's what you did, you tried to make them flow and be in between the straight lines. I was so pleased I had something to show him. Do you know what he said?'

I didn't expect it would be a compliment.

'Do you?' said William.

'No, but I don't expect it …' William interrupted me.

'I don't care what it looks like, I only want to know what it says.'

The edges of William's mouth turned down. I'd thought it would be something like that. I wondered if William's mother had gone to the school too.

'I could feel myself folding up, sort of creaking inside, I felt a door was going to slam shut inside me. I had got a silver star for this, not a gold one, but silver was the next best. He must have been able to see that. The teacher had stuck it on the fucking page.' He held up his hand, 'I'm sorry.'

'It's ok.'

'I tried to speak, but I couldn't get the words out, I was stumbling over them and I knew my dad was getting annoyed about that. I wanted to say: But they're just letters, they aren't words, they're just the letters I've been practising. Couldn't he see that? He must see that. "But what does it say?" he said. He'd tilt his head and raise his eyebrows at me and nod. "What does it say William?" My hands were tight little balls at the end of my arms, like in a cartoon. I could feel I was on the edge of crying. He was supposed to be pleased and he wasn't. It was happening again, it was all going wrong again. Other children's parents weren't like this. The other children didn't get this. It was all shit again, like the shit sandwiches, I couldn't spread butter on bread but I could make my letters flow. One of the nuns looked over at my dad, they looked at each

other, I looked at my letters. Then my dad said it was time to go home.'
William shrugged his shoulders, pinched his nose between his thumb
and forefinger, put his hand on the arm of the chair.

'I couldn't concentrate. I liked doing the letters at school, I liked drawing, but I couldn't concentrate.' He shut his eyes for a moment, then
turned his chair, looked at the knots on the walls. 'Sometimes I'll have
a creative idea, start to try to draw an image, make something, it will
happen by chance, spontaneous, I feel myself become interested, but
almost immediately I shut it down.' He turned back to me. 'The children
I was at school with, their families weren't like mine, they weren't cowed
and shamed. If something happened to them, if one of them got winded
they asked for help. Their parents were interested in them. When my
dad came to school and saw our handwriting, there were other parents
there. Their parents were paying attention.' William rubbed his jaw.

I was aware of all the stories and memories gathering in the room
with us.

'I know I spent a lot of time alone in my room. I didn't understand
what was going on, but I knew I shouldn't make any noise because
that just made them angry. And the longer it went on, I don't know,
I changed, like I didn't know how to be me anymore. I'd hear my father
coming up the stairs, walking down the hall towards my room. When
I heard him, I would go quiet, if it was night I would see the shape of his
shadow blocking out the light from the hall. I would know he was there
and I would go very quiet. I wanted help. But I knew I should be quiet.
All I wanted was to be let out of my room, to be taken downstairs and
join in with the others. Yet at those moments, when he was there, I kept
absolutely silent. I didn't want him to come in and tell me off. I'd lie with
the blanket pulled up over me, just rolling my head from one side to
another. Sometimes I'd want to go for a wee, but I would just lie there,
it might be a cold morning and I would pee, all the warm pee, then cold
and stingy. No one came. I think if they came they wouldn't know where
I was anyway.'

He stopped, rubbed his eyes, looked at me. 'What does this sound
like to you? All these stories, banging my head against the bars? Saying
made-up names, singsong-like, over and over. I went into myself, I don't
know, I went somewhere, I went into that triangle. I went into a place
inside me through that triangle. It sounds pretty crazy doesn't it?'

'It sounds very uncomfortable,' I said. I thought of the way these early traumas had undermined William.

William grunted, 'It sounds pretty mad to me. Very uncomfortable, oh yes. And the more I went into it, the further I got from the smell of my bed, the horrible rubbery sheet, from all of it, from the shame, the worthlessness.' William puffed out his cheeks and exhaled a long breath. 'Well, something like that.'

'I'm glad you brought the triangle image.'

'I don't think I should have,' said William.

'I don't suppose you do.'

'I'm surprised I brought it.'

I nodded. We sat in silence. I felt the mood ease a little, I crossed my legs, then uncrossed them. My eyes settled on the foot of the couch. It was only then that I noticed that I hadn't straightened the blanket, or the pillows. I wondered if William had noticed? He hadn't said anything about it. I wondered if William noticed all of my inconsistencies. I worried about being picked up for making a mistake and sneaked a sideways look at the Van Gogh print. I looked away, back at my shoes. I was aware that I'd lost my train of thought and I thought perhaps I should say something.

'Are you working on any other pictures?'

William stared at me.

'You think I go home and work on pictures?' William leant forward. 'What do you think this is about?', his voice forceful, confrontational.

I thought I should make my thoughts plain.

'I think you went through something traumatic,' I said, attempting to recover myself, 'and that you never knew when it would end. In some ways it doesn't sound like it has ended.'

William sat back, his expression mocking.

'Me going through trauma? I can't take that in.'

'No,' I said, 'I don't think you can. That's what I mean about it not having ended.'

William gave me a quizzical cross-face look. We sat, quiet. Outside, a red kite called, lyrical, plaintive; it got no response. It called again.

'You think I went through something traumatic and that it hasn't ended? That I'm still in it?' asked William.

'Yes,' I said.

William nodded, not mocking now.

'I'm not sure if I see it.'

I nodded.

We were silent.

The kite called out again.

'Can you say something?' William asked, 'I think the silence is making me anxious, like I'm being judged.' I looked at him. I thought of William's father, of impending judgement. 'Well,' said William 'then I'll tell you something, I am reading about Freud.'

I raised my eyes.

'Ah ha!' said William, 'got you! I thought you'd be interested.'

'What got you to Freud?' I said, giving a small laugh.

'Amazon, a book came up in a category search,' said William; he seemed pleased with the reaction. 'It's interesting, long-winded, and dry too, but the thing it says is that there is no substitute for doing the work in psychotherapy. I was pleased to see that. What? Why are you looking like that?'

'I was wondering if you are emulating me?' I said.

William laughed.

'That's a good one,' he said, 'I'll give you that. I'm emulating you.' It was time to stop. He collected his things, gave a short laugh and left.

Chapter 7

Ireland, September 1972

A knock on the door interrupted the sound of chalk hammering on the blackboard.

'Yes,' said Father Clevin, his sharp nasal tone loud, impatient, his chalk-holding hand suspended mid-air; he turned his head to see a school master come into the classroom, he lowered his hand. Father Clevin stepped from the platform, they met by the door and conferred.

At the back of the classroom, where a large faded map of the world covered up peeling paintwork, two boys caught each other's attention. They knew to be careful, they didn't want Father Clevin to catch them.

'Ask him his name,' said one.

'Ask him where he comes from,' said the other.

A short loud nasal laugh came from Father Clevin.

They were sat behind William who was copying fractions from the blackboard. A finger jabbed his shoulder. William glanced towards Father Clevin, saw he was still in conversation, then turned to find a ginger-haired boy inches from his face.

'Where do you come from?' asked the boy.

'What?' said William, he smiled, then said quietly, 'Leicester.'

'Westah,' said the boy. His friend sniggered and gave a mocking look.

'What's your name?'

'William, William Smith.'

'Wiwiam Smiff,' said the boy.

The classroom door shut.

'Quiet,' ordered Father Clevin scanning the room. 'Quiet Smith, concentrate on your work. Don't distract the other boys. We work in my class. I want good marks here. Is that clear?'

'Yes Father,' said William.

When class ended William turned to speak to the boys. He didn't mind that they'd poked fun at him. He hoped he might share the joke with them and that they could go to tea together. Standing, he lifted the lid of his hinged desk and collected his books.

'That was close,' he said, smiling, 'can I come to tea with you?'

The boys looked at each other.

'No,' said the first. 'We're not having tea with you Wiwiam. You better go back to Westah for your tea.' They sniggered and moved past him, past the desks and out of the classroom. William followed, the other boys were now already ahead of him and had split into groups. William hadn't found a way to fit in with any of them. He walked, following in their wake as they crossed the cold twilit road and headed to the dining room. In the hall, noise swelled: waves of conversations, bursts of laughter, strange accents, the clatter of trays and cutlery and the scraping of plates.

He hung back in the queue waiting his turn, listening, his thumb felt against the edge of the chipped tray. The noise in the hall marked a frontier to friendship that he couldn't find a way to cross. He breathed in the thick smell of the place, heavy and damp. The queue moved quickly. The tea-lady gave him baked beans, fish fingers from a vast oven tray, and a slice of white bread and margarine. He thanked her and took his tray to one of the long tables. A few boys were gathered at the other end, one of them looked at him, William smiled, the boy gave an indifferent look and turned back to his group and their conversation. William looked down at his food.

William, eleven now, had been at school for two weeks. He had been worried and excited about going, at first there had been something of an adventure about it. For a start, they had flown there, his mother, father, and Graham. His father told him that wouldn't happen again.

'We're only coming with you this once William. After that you can fly out with Graham,' said his father, 'he knows the ropes. But we'll come out this time, get your uniform, settle you in.'

His father told him they wouldn't be staying long. His father had people he wanted to visit while he was over in Ireland.

'I better get something out of it for me,' his father had said. William was aware that Graham didn't seem happy to be going back.

William looked at the beans and pushed some on to his fork. He thought the margarine tasted horrible, but ate it, knowing it was the last meal until the morning. He ate the tepid unappetising food, disliking the way the beans and fish fingers went together in his mouth. He thought of home. His brother Graham was somewhere about the school, but being three years older than William he was in the senior school and didn't spend much time with him. Graham knew that William was finding things difficult, that the other boys laughed at his accent. He wished Graham would come and find him.

After tea the boys would disperse to activities before it was time for prep. At the start of the term William hadn't known what activity to pick, it seemed everything he tried to sign up to was already full. He'd ended up being given library time.

Leaving the dining room he crossed the road back to the main school block, his books still under his arm, and climbed the worn stone stairs to the library. A tall elderly priest was coming down the stairs towards him.

'Are you alright boy?' asked the priest.

'Yes Father,' said William. The unexpected interest took him by surprise.

'Are you going to the library?' asked the priest.

'Yes Father,' said William.

'Very good,' said the priest and he carried on past him down the stairs.

Leaning on the heavy iron catch he pushed open the stiff black wooden door and entered the hushed room. The library felt neglected, lifeless, as if he was stepping into a place that most of the school had forgotten. He put his books down on a table by the window. It was darker outside. He could see his blank reflection looking back at him in the leaded window panes, a dull version of himself, lonely, disengaged. There were magazines on a round table, he'd flicked through them several times already. On the end wall were pictures of boys from years gone by. He'd looked at them before, trying to pick out his father, who had assured him there were several pictures of himself dotted around the school. William hadn't found one.

He killed time amongst the bookshelves. He hadn't found anything he was interested in, he hadn't worked out the library at all. There were some poetry books and then there were bound volumes of obscure journals and some encyclopaedias. He leafed through them, but nothing took his interest. There were two other boys sitting apart at a table, one appeared to be doing his homework. William nodded to them, he wondered if they were lost souls like him. One of them nodded back, the other boy stuck to his task, head propped on his hand, his pen busy on the paper in front of him.

'I didn't want to go to boarding school, and I knew Graham didn't want to go back. When we were at the airport having a sandwich waiting for the flight, I could see Graham's face, he was sitting there just staring at the ground. He wanted to leave and go to art school but my father would have none of it. Everything was strange, weird. The priests who taught us, the monks in their black robes. The endless church, Mass, compulsory confession, I didn't like it at all.'

'This was the school your father had gone to?'

'Yes, he thought a lot of the place, was always telling me how lucky I was. My youngest daughter has just gone to boarding school, we let her, in England. She wanted to go, we'd never have suggested it. I didn't feel that happy about her going away but she was set on it. It's different for her. She's having a good time, the social life, the sports, it all works for her. She isn't sitting on her own, unhappy, in a library every night staring at maps.'

I nodded. William looked at me.

'You're always nodding,' said William. 'The priests were always nodding. You'd have fit right in.'

Ireland, September 1972

William reached for the atlas again. He sat at his table and leafed through the oversized pages trying to find his home in England. He wondered how it was at home. He imagined his mother reading her Greek, her endless hobby, his father might be back from golf now, would it be lighter there? Did the sun set there first? He wasn't sure. He had looked in the library for Greek books, had thought of trying to write a line from a Greek myth home to his mother. He liked the Greek myths—Odysseus, Theseus, Jason and the Argonauts.

He found Greece in the atlas. He looked at the islands, he thought of being with his mother, with his family, all of them on holiday. He imagined going to Greece, playing, exploring the Acropolis. He missed home, he didn't like being away, though he knew being back at home wouldn't be right either. He couldn't understand any of it—unhappy at school, unhappy at home. Home wasn't here; he didn't want to be here, alone. He could feel the homesick feeling rising in his stomach and chest. He didn't want to have those feelings now, he didn't want to get upset.

At the airport his father had said he would soon get into the swing of things, make great friends.

'Don't look so worried William, it's off-putting, put a smile on your face. Throw yourself into it, that's the way to make friends and get on. I mean look at Graham,' said his father. 'If he went to art school he'd lose all his friends, right Graham?'

Graham looked up, opened his mouth.

'I would, Dad, but I could stay in touch with them, and I could get on with my art,' said Graham.

'Get on with your art? You think you're Michelangelo? Well you're not. Art?' scoffed his father. 'Do you have the art of putting a smile on this one's face?' He pointed his folded newspaper at William. 'Because I don't. That's the art that counts. William, you're putting me off my tea. Go for a walk around, the pair of you. Come back when they call the flight.'

'We could fly anywhere from here, Dad,' said William, 'we could go on holiday.'

'What?' retorted his father, 'life's not a holiday William. You've just had a holiday, a long holiday, I think you spent most of the time up in your room. It's time to get on with yourself now. Ridiculous.' His father glared at their mother, who, with a turn of the head, let his look slide past her. He picked up his paper, looked at his watch, and turned back to the crossword, muttering to himself.

Graham got up and walked away. William looked at his mother, then followed Graham across the airport.

Now he was here, in Ireland. He'd have to go back to his house soon, he couldn't go back looking upset, the boys would pick up on it. He tried to jolt himself out of the mood before the feelings got the better of him, something to distract himself, he put the atlas away. He looked at the shelves, trying to find something that would catch his attention, anything. It wasn't going to work. He caught sight of his reflection in the window. Put a smile on your face, his father would say. He gathered his things together and left.

Leaving by the library's side door he stepped into a wide empty hall. He could feel the edge of the cold night air, it had the run of the place. He pulled his jacket tight, thought about Greece again.

The portraits of previous headmasters looked down on him, alone, his books pulled under one arm. He walked the length of the hall. With each step he felt the undulations of the floor tiles, worn down, they curved, uneven. His father would have walked this corridor. He took in the thick smell of polish. He wondered if his father remembered the smell. He didn't think you'd forget it.

His history classroom was on his right, the door ajar, the lights still on. He listened to hear if Father O'Malley was there. He didn't get too close to the door. He turned back, retraced his steps, walked back past the classrooms, past the library and descended the wide stone staircase again. The building was silent but for his footsteps and the occasional sound of boys shouting to each other from outside. From deep within the school a bell began to ring—the prep bell. He walked to the side staircase, past the staff room, the lingering smell of pipe tobacco, the telephone kiosk. He thought about calling home but knew it wasn't allowed. He made his way back to his house, glad at least that it wasn't raining. It would be warmer, though his heart sank at the thought of being there; being lonely by himself was one thing, being ignored in the common room was worse.

He walked past the chapel, making out the dim-lit stained glass, the blue edge of the Blessed Mary's gown. Was anyone in there now? Were they finishing confession? He didn't like the confessionals, they were claustrophobic and the horrible incense smell was overpowering. He picked up his pace, skirted the edge of the main school playing field and made his way back to the road.

Inside the house, in the prep room a couple of boys perched on the black iron radiator, others were sitting down at their desks. They all seemed to fit in, some of them local boys, some from towns further away; they all had different accents. William was the only boy from England, and Graham too. At the back of his school diary he had drawn a grid of seventy-seven squares. Fifty-three days until the Christmas holiday; with deliberate care he shaded out yesterday. He heard movement, the prep room door swung shut, Father Michael had come in.

'Good evening boys,' said Father Michael. 'Away from the radiator now, get to your desks. Get on now.'

The boys obeyed. For a few moments a chorus of sound built, desk drawers being opened and shut, chairs scraped on linoleum. Each night they would go through this, the noise building, a prep-room crescendo. William liked it, he looked furtively towards the boy at the next desk. The boy looked at him and dropped his books with a thud. William smiled, the boy raised his eyes. From behind him he heard another boy snigger. He wished he could become part of it. He couldn't understand why everyone was so unfriendly.

'Quiet now,' said Father Michael and that was the end of it. In the silence William felt his discomfort stir again, he felt it in his chest, he couldn't concentrate, he sat grappling with his feelings. He took out his writing paper.

> Dear Mum and Dad,
> I need to come home to England, I am so unhappy here. Please come and rescue me urgently as soon as you read this, otherwise I think I will die.
> Love

He imagined them getting his letter. He concentrated on the image of his mother and father reading it and wanting to come and get him. He pictured receiving a letter from them by return.

> *Dear Son,*
> *We got your letter today and we are coming to take you home right*
> *now. Don't worry.*
> *Love*

Father Michael pushed his chair back and stood, the noise interrupted William's reverie. The priest walked slowly round the room, he looked down at their work as he did. William tried to move his letter out of sight and open a textbook, but it was too late. Father Michael picked the letter up.

'You should be doing your homework William, write letters home in your spare time. What's this?' William felt his panic leap, he feared he was going to read it out to the rest of the boys, he knew some of the priests could be cruel like that. But Father Michael had a sympathetic side to him, he gave William his letter back. 'Concentrate on your work, that's my advice. Ok William?' said Father Michael.

'Yes Father,' said William, relieved. He put the letter in his desk drawer, took out his maths book and turned to the fractions he'd copied earlier. Wiwiam fwom Westah.

Each morning there was a break from lessons at 11am when the boys would return to their houses to change their schoolbooks. Then they would check to see what post had arrived; letters from home were special. It had been four days since he'd written to his parents, the letter Father Michael had seen. It was probably too soon for a reply but nonetheless he scanned the common room table. He tried to look at the envelopes casually at first, it was a trick he played on himself, a way of restraining his hope. There was a letter, he could see his father's writing, his spirits lifted. Picking it up he sat in one of the tatty armchairs and tore through the envelope; a short message stared up at him.

> *Dear Son,*
> *Stop sending us letters full of emotional blackmail. It upsets us.*
> *Love*
> *Mum*

William slowed to a stop, horrified, shamed. The common room was louder now, soon they would all have to return to the school buildings for lessons. He placed the letter back in the envelope, he sat, still. He didn't know what to do with himself.

———•———

'It upset them? I had the letter in my hand, I was horrified. I didn't want anyone to come and see. Not that they would have. I can't tell you how I felt. I really thought they'd written to tell me they were on their way. That it was over. And they said I was blackmailing them. I've never forgotten that.' William leant forward in his chair. 'It was shame, I felt ashamed. Love mum, there wasn't much love in it.'

I felt for William.

William stared at me. 'Do you know what that kind of shock is like?' I looked back at him, at the anger and hurt. I thought of my own experiences, injustices, wounds. 'Do you?' repeated William, demanding. His eyes wide, expectant.

'I don't know if I do,' I said.

'No,' said William. 'Well it was terrible. I didn't know what to do with myself. This acute feeling of shame and guilt. And I had to carry on. I had to get my books, go back to lessons. I felt empty. Somehow I had let myself hope that they would come for me, I'd let myself believe it, it was like a door slamming on me, another door. I felt it would be better if I was dead.'

I was aware of William revealing more of his story, more of the contexts of himself. I tried not to do anything to disrupt the process. William looked out of the window, then shut his eyes, rubbed his chin, tapped his index finger against his cheek. 'Of course they wouldn't come. If I'd been some other child with different parents they'd have come and got me. If my daughter sent a letter like that home from her school I would be there to get her before the return post. And I'd let myself think they'd do the same.' He stared across at me. I looked back at him. I thought: this is how it had developed for William, one vulnerability and weakness stacked upon another. 'Do you think I'm overstating it?' asked William.

'I don't think you saw it coming,' I said. William turned back to the window, then back to me.

'I had let myself believe they would come. I remember it like it just happened, me sitting in the chair in the common room. The people around me all noisy, getting on with things, having a good time. They didn't get letters like that. I stuffed it into my pocket, later I tore it into tiny pieces, I didn't want anyone finding it and shaming me. I don't know how I got through the rest of the day, the days that followed. There was no escape. It must have been obvious, in my body language. I felt worthless, like I did at home. I didn't deserve anything.' He closed his eyes and put his hand to the side of his head, he looked like he was touching a bruise.

'I think it felt like a terrible rejection,' I said. I wondered as I said it if that word was appropriate.

William looked at me, silent.

'Looking back on it, I think I was in quite a bad way,' said William. 'I don't know how I got through it. I drifted through the rest of that day, the days that followed. I couldn't concentrate on things. I was in a state. If I became interested in anything, something in an art lesson, I would feel I should drop it straightaway. Everything was forbidden to me. I didn't deserve anything. I felt guilty. Other boys could write home and get help. I didn't deserve that. I was worthless.' He looked at me. 'Rejection. That is what it was, another rejection. You know when I first came to see you, I remember I checked that this time would be ok with you, do you remember?' said William. I nodded, I did. 'You said this was my time. I really liked you saying that. This is my time,' said William.

'Yes,' I said, gesturing an apology. 'But it is time to stop.'

William nodded, gathered his things and left.

Ireland, October 1973

There in the school, weighed down by shame, rejection, and worthlessness William sank further into himself. Days ticked by slowly, the weekends were interminable, he was scared to write home, scared to call home. He felt rebuked by the mail when it was spread out on the common room table, scared of getting another angry letter. He was scared of himself and the reactions he provoked in his home, he was intimidated by the monks in their heavy black robes. He went through the routine of school life, the chapel, the meals, the lessons. He was alone and unhappy, and it was all he deserved, he had upset his parents and been put in his place again. There was no getting away from it.

On the way to classes, in the dining hall, he listened to the voices around him, all the strange rolling accents, some from the north, some from the south, he had learned there were differences. The different voices went up and down, he copied them to himself. Their sing-song tones ran through his head, they didn't sound shamed and rejected.

Reflecting William's mood, the weather turned, dark clouds rolled in one following the other. It rained for a week, then another. Life went on at the school, day by crossed-out day, the routines became more familiar, only wetter. Then things took an unexpected turn.

William was called for rugby trials and was one of the boys who made the squad. It turned out that he was good at sport and he was selected to play for the school. When he got into the team the boys stopped taking the mickey out of him, they stopped trying to make him say things they could laugh at. To his surprise he discovered, as he ran, as he opened his hands again to catch the muddy ball that span towards him, this time from the left, not the right, that he was fitting in. At the same time, he made subtle alterations to his voice, he already knew how to copy their accents.

In the rugby team he saw that there was one boy who stood out. Off the field William watched the way the boy carried himself. He started to mimic him, carefully copying his style without being too blatant about it. William and he were both picked to play centres in the next match. The boy was conceited and didn't notice he was being copied, but he found himself taking to William. He started to think that they were quite alike.

Alternating, on Saturdays and Wednesdays they played matches against other schools, home one week, away the next. They won more than they lost. They were not the strongest school team in the county but not the weakest either and their partnership in the centres was one of the strengths of the team. They ran straight, they didn't miss tackles, they had good hands and could pass the ball. The games teacher said if he had a few more like them they'd win the school league.

The other boy was popular, the leader of a small group, boys who had known each other for years and who were at school together before coming here. Gradually, William fitted in with them outside of rugby and changes started to follow. He no longer ate tea alone, he was part of a group now; at mealtimes they shuffled up and made space for him at their table. William could see there was some envy from one of the other boys, could see he had inadvertently pushed some of them aside. He didn't worry about it—as long as he was fitting in there was no need to worry. And it didn't stop there: now William was picked for other teams. He wrote home to tell his parents. William had become one of a gang, close to the leader. There was a marked improvement in his daily life, he knew he had put on a mask, that what the other boys and the rest of the school saw wasn't really him, but he didn't mind. It wasn't the same as being himself, it was an act, but daily life was better than it was. Sometimes he forgot to cross out the days at the back of his diary. When he remembered, he shook his head with disbelief, while the boy beside him showed him his latest aeroplane drawings.

'This is what I meant by emulating,' said William. 'Like I said when I first came to see you. I copied the successful boys and it created a layer of insulation around me, and I thought if I can keep this up I might be able to get through to the holidays. It was instinctive, strange, but it wasn't really me, it was a system I was using, and it was like it was just there waiting for me all along, it protected me, but it wasn't me. I would sometimes hear it in my voice, the way I was speaking, the falseness.'

'You were fitting in,' I said, not sure if that was quite the right way to put it.

'No,' said William, raising his right hand from where it had been settled on the arm of the chair. 'You've got that wrong. That's what I'm trying to say. I wasn't fitting in. It was this other me. I was emulating them.'

'Yes,' I said, 'that's what I meant.'

'Was it? You say something like that, and I think you don't understand what I'm telling you. It makes me think that I might be making a mistake coming here.' William looked at me and then turned away. I felt put in my place. I didn't say anything else; it was a delicate moment. William shuffled his feet.

Outside, two jackdaws called back and forth. I listened to them, chastened, they seemed to know how to talk to each other. After a while William continued.

'That wasn't me. It was like I'd been put somewhere else, this other version of me was doing things, emulating. Making things predictable, safe. I was just getting through it.'

William looked at me, dubious, then he placed his hand back on the arm of the chair.

Chapter 8

Ireland, December 1973

Finally the Christmas holiday is less than a week away and William will soon be returning to England. Six squares stand in his way and he doesn't bother to shade them all in. A lightness starts to come over him, he thinks about home, being away from the school, with its rolling accents and horrible food. He thinks of his voice sounding normal again and that thought surprises him. His voice, not having to roll his words, an inkling of dropping the act of himself. Not having to keep his eye on everything and everyone around him, being himself again. Being himself again? He isn't quite sure what that means now. Around him the other boys read books, draw pictures of aeroplanes mid dog fights, there's not much homework to do. William feels secretive; half an idea, if that, occurs to him that at some point in the term he turned away from himself. He has never spoken about that at confession. They don't know you're lying, the priests say they do but they don't, not when you know to keep secrets like he does.

William feels he has lived a lie, become this other him, and the boys and the monks don't seem to have noticed at all. Why would they? They never knew him before. Who remembers Wiwiam from Westah now?

And it's curious but he can see he has hardly noticed it either, he has just become this other him. He has been fixed on copying the other boys and making things predictable and safe. He hasn't allowed himself to think about the other him, the him he used to see reflected in the empty dark library windows. The memories shame him. Father Mackenzie knew something of it; he wonders if Father Mackenzie remembers. The other William that has been carefully shut away. He isn't quite sure how he did it, he supposes that if he didn't let himself see it, then no one else would. He starts to feel disoriented, a twinge of alarm, as he lets himself acknowledge this other crossed-out story. He steadies himself, he knows no one would know how to read it. All the feelings he used to cross out and hide behind meticulously shaded pencil lines. He shuts the diary and places it amongst his books, cautiously lifts his eyes, and tilting his head up just enough and incrementally, he scans the room. Father MacKenzie is absorbed in writing their termly reports, 'Be quiet boys and I might say you behaved yourselves.' Everyone is quiet, reading, writing, drawing, there might not be much work going on, but they are quiet. He fixes himself on the quiet of the prep room.

The boy on his right is methodically shading a picture of an aeroplane, he has drawn them all term, William thinks he must have seen squadrons. Soon he will be on a plane flying back to England, that's something, his parents will meet him at the airport. He is going home, he imagines not having to come back again, which makes his eyes widen. Being in his own bedroom, not having to sleep in the dormitory. Home, being warm, maybe they will have got central heating while he's been away. He wants to be away from this cold wet place.

He has been measured and on guard all the time. He never knew he would be so good at mimicry. Now he will be free of it. He will get in a taxi and go to the airport and leave it behind. He has kept all of these thoughts hidden away, even from himself. He looks at one of his hands, then the other, this other him. He thinks he will have to be careful otherwise he might give himself away, act differently and the boys will see through him and he'll be back at square one. He'll be Wiwiam from Westah again, stammering, feeble, lost and alone. He mustn't let that happen.

'I was nervous, and excited I suppose,' said William. 'But I don't know what I was thinking of. They didn't come to meet us at the airport. We got the train, then a taxi. As soon as I stepped into my home I was back in that atmosphere.' William paused and turned his chair back towards the window. 'I could feel the mood of the place. It seemed to be waiting for me on the gravel. It had been there all along.'

Leicester, December 1973

In the hallway they hung up their coats, William asked questions, he was looking for Flo. His mother said she'd forgotten his questions, she said she'd not missed them. It was a joke, a bit like a joke at school, but it weighed on him. She told them to take their cases up to their rooms and then come down for supper. As they turned to leave, Flo appeared at the top of the stairs, William's mood lifted at the sight of her.

William had fixed his mind on being home, with his mother, on the thought of her wanting to be with him; he had hung the image in front of him. Now, as they gathered together in the kitchen, he can feel the effort he's making to keep his idealised version in place.

They talked—him, Graham, and Flo—but his mother appeared indifferent. She'd made soup and William helped her carry bowls and bread to the table. William told her how delicious it looked, told her how awful the food at the school tasted, she waved him away and rested the ladle at the side of the pan. She said she didn't suppose it was that bad, and anyway, he had gone on about that enough in his letters. William thought of his homesick letter and the reply he received. He wondered if she remembered that letter. He felt ashamed and wasn't sure what to say. He ran his hand over the grain of the table, pressed his palm into the wood like he did to the wood of his desk in the prep room at school. The four of them sat in silence. Flo sighed, said 'this is fun.' William looked at her. She pulled a face at him and stirred her soup. William started to ask her a question but then stopped himself. Flo pulled a funny face, asked him to say more. William didn't.

Flo started to tell a story about school, she told them she was going to boarding school next year. She was excited. It was in England. William was relieved it wasn't in Ireland. He was about to say something when he noticed his mother was reaching for her book. He dipped bread into his bowl. He had let himself think it would be different at home, that he was going somewhere that wanted him, somewhere he would know how to be him again. As the butter melted on his bread he watched his ideas coming apart.

He ate the bread and soup, concentrating so his spoon didn't touch the side of the bowl, he didn't want to disturb the peace. He had the curious sense of feeling he hadn't really come home, stirring the half-thought into the soup. Here he thought he would be free of the performance of school but he wasn't, he was still the other him; he stirred that thought into the soup too. He lifted his eyes and glanced at his mother, who didn't notice, she was in her books again. William allowed himself to watch her, he recognised her expression, he knew she was concentrating on a particular word. William wondered where his mother had put his other mother, the mother who used to be soppy with him. He wondered if she knew. He wanted to ask her but didn't. He stirred his soup.

They all heard the front door open, their father call out from the hall.

'Are the boys back? Ruining the peace already are you? Eh?' William's father came into the kitchen, he rubbed his hands together for warmth. 'And eating all of my soup I suppose.' His father looked at them both and smiled. 'Graham, William, shake my hand, it's good to see you.'

'Hello Dad,' said Graham.

'Your hands are soft Graham, is that what all your art does to you? William, you're looking a bit better.' William felt himself bask in his father's comment. His father tore a piece of bread from William's plate, dipped it in the soup and ate it.

'Have you been playing golf Dad?' said William. His father popped a piece of bread into his mouth.

'Hole in one eh,' said his father, chewing the bread. 'So, when are you both going back then?' asked his father walking out of the room. With that, William began counting down the days.

His father spent his time working, or at the golf course; if it was too dark or wet to play he still preferred to be there, drinking with his friends, to being at home. At his mother's suggestion—William over-heard their conversation—his father arranged a Christmas Eve game of golf for William, Graham, and himself. William was unsettled, he couldn't concentrate or relax. He was always watching what went on around him. With Flo and Graham he joined their attempt at a 1,000-piece jigsaw puzzle, but in his hands the pieces would not join up. His mood remained agitated. Flo said he was worrying the pieces. William laughed, said 'No I'm not.' Flo pulled a face at him, and said 'No I'm not,' mimicking the strange Irish accent he'd come home with. But she was right, he was worrying, nervous, he could feel the state of it in him all of the time.

'That's the piece I was looking for,' said Flo.

'Oh, yes, sorry,' said William.

'I'm going to change your name to Sorry,' said Flo.

He worried about playing golf with his father. He knew it would be competitive, that his father would want to beat them and that he'd mock their loose shots. When his father was out, he took a golf club from the garage and practised on the common, telling himself to relax. But he needn't have worried—at the last minute his father cancelled to play with his friends instead. Even then, William didn't know if he was relieved or disappointed. He heard himself say 'Oh no that's alright Dad,' then worried he should have said something else, had he said it wrong? Should he have sounded more disappointed? He was left alone in the hallway balancing his feelings, his father having already walked away. He knew he was wary of reacting in a way that his father would dislike.

He watched Graham's persistent attempts to speak about going to art school. He could see his father didn't want to have that conversation again. William worried there would be some almighty row. He went for walks on his own and he spent time in his room; the elephant curtains had gone now. He lay in bed at night, his door ajar, and watched for the shadows his mother and father cast down the hallway as they went up to their room. He found he couldn't fall asleep until they had gone to bed. Each night he waited for them to turn off the landing light and for the house to go dark. Only then did he settle.

———•———

'No, it's here, er … hyperarousal, is that the right word?' said William, looking up from his phone.

'Yes, I think it might be.'

'What does it mean?' said William. 'I mean I know what it means, but what do you think of me saying that?'

'Do you mean does it apply to you?' I asked. William said nothing. I tried again. 'Where did you find it?'

'I was looking into trauma, into PTSD. I found it in a description of an army veteran. Hyperarousal was the word they used. You must know about PTSD?'

'Yes. I thought about trauma too,' I said, deflecting the point a little. I didn't want us to become mired in the language of psychological diagnoses. I didn't think of William as a diagnosis. I thought of his problems as stemming from contexts, from things that happened to him that he hadn't yet caught up with and had a chance to process, from early traumas that had left him vulnerable to further traumas.

'It's me. I think it's the right word,' said William. He was quiet for a while before continuing. 'Going home, the holidays. I wasn't sure what I had been looking forward to. God it's a puzzle to me.' His blank stare settled on me. 'I went for walks, I was at a loose end. Whatever I did I ended up in my room thinking about going back to school. I couldn't really engage with my family.'

'It sounds like your sister picked up on things.'

'Flo, yes, she's perceptive, she did, but I couldn't engage with her.'

'You couldn't flow,' I said. William smiled.

'No,' he said, 'I couldn't flow. That's quite funny. But I couldn't, I was too tense, too, I don't know … in myself. One day I started doodling in my room and before I knew it I was marking out another grid and counting down the days again. I didn't want to go back. I wanted to be in a home where you were wanted, but that wasn't where I was. I couldn't relax.'

'It makes me think about you asking me about the word hyperarousal,' I said.

'Meaning?' said William

'Well it made me think that there are times when you relax here.'

'What makes you say that?'

'You asking the question,' I said.

'It's not the first time I've asked a question,' William shot back, his finger starting to tap on the arm of his chair.

'No,' I said, wishing I'd kept my mouth shut.

Leicester, January 1973

Square by square, the holidays came to an end. One day, William was sat in his room at home packing his suitcase; the next, he was unpacking it at school. When he did so, he unpacked his mother's white woollen cardigan, which he'd stolen from her room before he left. Now he hid it in the chest beside his bed in the dormitory. Each night he went to sleep cuddled up to it, inhaling the faint scent of his mother.

Chapter 9

Ireland, January 1973

He sat at his desk in the prep room looking at the grid in the back of his new term diary. He was back at square one. He felt the homesickness well up in him again, the anxious feeling. He pushed it down, it's not as bad this time. But it hasn't gone away, it seems to be a dull constant now, just shifted location from home back to school.

The boys he's become friends with are pleased to see him, oblivious to anything he is going through. He concentrates on becoming that version of himself that fits in; it's uncanny, but he feels himself transforming into the school him again, hears his voice change as he copies their accents. The more he lets himself lean into it, the more he becomes the school him. They think he is good at games, they don't know the half of it. Home is behind him now, and he accepts it, he is going to fit in with this now and make the best of it. This intention takes him through the remainder of the school year and most of the next.

———————

William settled his things on the table beside him, spreading his jacket flat across his knees.

'Have you ever worked with anyone like me before?' We looked at each other, I thought the question over.

'What makes you ask?'

'I want to check if you understand, if you know what we're doing? If you know where we are going? I have got all these questions going round and round,' said William.

'What questions?'

'I've told you about things that I didn't know I knew,' said William. 'But I wonder if you have worked with someone like me before. In your experience, how difficult a case am I?' I thought before replying. What could I say? I didn't want to start talking about William as a case.

'I think this is difficult,' I said, hoping I'd caught the right tone.

'I am very glad you've said that,' said William, nodding. He looked relieved. He sank back into his chair, it reclined with him. 'I can't see it, I can feel it is difficult, but I can't see it. I wanted to know if you could. It's strange, I am relieved by you saying that. I can feel myself welling up.' He broke off, leant forward and stretched his shoulders back. 'It's very uncomfortable too.' I thought he looked emotional. William closed his eyes and looked down at the rug between us. When he looked up again his face was more composed.

'You felt yourself welling up?'

'Yes, and as soon as I feel it I try to shut it down,' replied William. 'It's like a reflex. I can't help it.'

'No.'

'The feelings start coming up and I,' he broke off and gestured with his hands, 'I shut them down straight away. But it's you saying that this is difficult. You saying that connected with me. I could feel it. I think I want that, but it scares me. I don't know what to make of it. I shut it down. Why is that?' William gripped his jacket, his hands pressed into his knees. He looked at me, then looked away.

'I think these are difficult things, perhaps scary too,' I said.

'I feel ashamed,' said William.

'You said you felt your feelings well up when I said it was difficult,' I said.

'Yes,' said William. 'That went straight through me. In a way that doesn't normally happen. Why is that?' We looked at each other.

'I think it's a different side of you, not a side that gets very much attention.'

'It probably doesn't get any attention,' said William.

'No,' I said, 'but I think you working like this is an attempt to find a way to give it attention now, speaking about the memories. Perhaps particularly these experiences of how you had to fit in, emulate as you say. I think that in the experience of fitting in, these feelings were put away, put in their place.'

'And now they well up?' said William.

'That might be right, yes.'

William was silent. He let go of his jacket and leant back in his chair.

'Well I feel better for it,' said William. 'But I fight it away as soon as I start to feel it happening, even though I know I feel better for it, and when I leave I'll flip. I'll attack myself.' He shook his head gently and looked at the Van Gogh print. I still regretted the picture being there, I felt I'd become allergic to it. Looking back at me, William said 'I remember in an art class we were shown a surrealist painting by Paul Nash, *The Menin Road*. Do you know it?' I shook my head. 'No? Well I was amazed by it. I had never seen anything like it. I was looking at it and I could feel the energy of my interest catch hold of me. I had the strange sense of being drawn out of myself by the picture. I wasn't emulating now, this was me looking back at the picture. I felt fascinated by it, and almost immediately I felt that I must drop it. It was like a voice in my head saying "This isn't for you. Other people can be interested in this. But not you." I felt a sense of shame and unease and I felt myself back away from the painting. I backed away from my interest, sneaked away from it and, I don't know, went further into myself. This wasn't for me, this was for other people.' He sat silent.

'I think there are these moments, when you don't react from the point of emulating and fitting in, moments when your own feelings well up spontaneously.'

'Yes,' William responded. 'But I shut them down straight away. There's no conversation about it, they are just shut away. I think that's the hyper-arousal. But it's strange how I remember that painting. I want more of it, but I'm not allowed it. What's that about?'

'That may be the difficulty we're talking about,' I said.

'Reacting to paintings like that, having feelings, that's all forbidden. I get angry with myself, I can't stop it. Those kinds of things are for other people.'

Ireland, January 1973

So he emulated. He knew it was a kind of act he was performing but nobody else seemed to notice. He copied the other boys and he did it expertly. He was like a spy in a novel who had forgotten he was a spy. It was hard to remember he was once Wiwiam from Westah; now he was at the heart of the group. He was in all the sports teams. He had become one of them. Everyone was convinced, but they didn't all like it.

William had become friends with the group leader, a consequence of which was that he had pushed another boy out into the sidelines. The boy nursed a grudge, he used to be first to join in, now he was an also-ran. He was offended by William—everything had been fine till he turned up. Over time his resentment and envy grew. William hadn't meant to cause him any offence, but that's how the boy felt it. The boy stewed on his feelings until one day he found an opportunity and started to complain to others in the group. At first they didn't pay him any attention. But the boy persevered. He commented to them about how William was mimicking their voices. He asked if they remembered Wiwiam from Westah? Some of them did. He gained their confidence and they started to listen. He commented on how everything had changed since William turned up, saying they had all been pushed aside to make way for him. This small group started to become focused on William and their envy of him, and one day they ambushed him as they all walked back from games and a confrontation ensued.

'Why are you always copying us?' The boy with the grudge was right in his face, his eyes wide, mouth open.

'Eh?' the boy persisted. William wasn't sure what to say, he hadn't seen this coming. 'You're always copying us,' said the boy, 'everything we do, why do you do that? Eh?'

William was caught off guard. For the briefest of moments he thought it might pass over, that it would turn out to be a joke, but the moment came to nothing, the boy wasn't joking. The attack was so quick and unexpected that it caught William out. There and then everything unravelled, the boy's accusation went straight to the truth of the matter. The emulatory shield that only seconds ago had been so reliable and protective dissolved as though it had never been there. William felt his shame rise up and envelop him, he felt they could see right into the secret shamed internal core of him. William looked to the group leader to support him. All it would take would be some comment from him, but the boy didn't look back. William realised this had been plotted. The accusing boy smelt victory and stepped even closer into William, following up with the questions and accusations, and before long it was over and William was cast out of the group.

The boys walked off, leaving him alone by a corner flag on the edge of one of the playing fields. He could hear them laughing, taking the mickey out of him and his voice as they walked away.

He was horrified, he could hardly walk. He didn't know where to walk to. Suddenly the whole place felt hostile again. There was no sanctuary, no place for him on their table in the dining hall. In the privacy of the prep room he blocked out squares again in the back of his diary. His pencil went over them with such focus that it sometimes went right through the paper.

He made it to the end of the term. He went home for the Christmas break and asked not to be sent back. His parents were having none of it. He went for long walks on his own. Before he knew it he was sitting at the airport again waiting for his flight to be called. At school he was alone again, he dropped out of the sports teams and his school work suffered. He spent a lot of time walking around the school grounds, unable to face his reflection in the library windows. He felt there was only one thing left open to him, he would try again. He wrote home for help. He let himself believe that this time they would take pity on him, feel his need for them and their protection, see it in his words. He tried again to conceive of himself as fitting back into a world in which children were wanted and safe. He tried to block out his doubts. When he sent the letter, he concentrated only on the idea that he would be rescued, that this would all be over and he would be free to go home.

He wrote:

> Dear Mum and Dad,
> I am very unhappy. I have no friends and I need you to come and take me away from this school.
> I really need you now as I have nowhere else to turn.
> Love

To his surprise he received a quick response, a letter from home, his father was coming. William cannot believe his eyes. His father was coming to get him.

Chapter 10

William lurked, waiting at the back of the class. Across from him Father Michael's robes swayed as he stepped from the blackboard saying something about Gabriel and the Annunciation that William didn't catch, because just then the sound of the hand bell jangling in the corridor triggered an irresistible wave of noise, of foot-scraping and chair-shifting, of desks being opened and shut, and in that instant William thought he might rise from his desk like a bird and sing with joy.

He ran his fingers over the scratched grain of the desk for the last time and, without thinking to pick up his books, went to push his way into the queue pressing to leave the room. Then he was out, jostling with boys emptying from classrooms and near-jogging down the corridor, past the notice boards, out through the main arch and into the clutches of the mean January wind, free from the boys dispersing in groups across footpaths, free from the school.

Before he got to the car park he recognised the tall figure coming towards him. At first he thought his father was pleased to see him, but as they got closer it struck him that his father was pleased to see the school, not him. His father looked down at William before turning to the chapel and the main school block.

'It's something, this place, isn't it,' said his father. He tutted. 'Hello William.'

'Hello Dad.'

They shook hands and for a moment stood stiffly together surveying the ivy-covered stone buildings, William bidding them a last goodbye.

'Let's go around this way,' said his father, 'by the playing fields.' His father pushed William's elbow and they started to walk.

'Ok,' said William, his hands and his hopes pressed into his pockets.

At a measured pace his father led them around the school grounds. William began to feel uneasy, every step was taking him further from his wish that his father would tell him to get his suitcase and put it in the back of the car. That was the thought he'd hung nearly every waking moment on since his father's letter arrived.

'This place hasn't changed at all,' said his father, 'though the road is busier. You were more cut off in my day.'

Past the chapel, his father pointed them to a bench beneath two leafless wind-bent trees that overlooked the sports field. There they sat. Away from them, three boys were practising drills. Two of them took it in turn to shoot at the goal while the goalkeeper tried to block their shots. His father pulled the collars of his overcoat together and leant forward, absorbed in watching them. A white ball shot across the pitch.

'Good shot that, eh. Very good,' he clapped the boys who were too far away to hear him. 'You should be out there practising William, are you on the hockey team?'

'No, Dad,' said William. He wasn't on any team now.

'It's a shame, you'll regret it later. God I wish I still played. Just to have the chance to play on a pitch like that. Good shot! You wouldn't want to be in the way of that ball.' William realised then that he was a spare part in his father's reflections. His father had come to watch hockey practice, not to rescue him. While the goalkeeper retrieved the ball, the outfield players switched places. Now his father turned to look at William, who could not bring himself to lift his eyes from the patch of worn grass below his sorry scuffed shoes. His father told William to look him in the eye. William forced himself to look up.

Taking the glove from his right hand his father reached within his coat. To his horror, William saw the letter he'd sent home reappear in front of him. His father held it out before him, proof of guilt. William stared at it, shamed: Mr and Mrs Smith … loopy writing.

'These letters have got to stop William. Do you have any idea what it does to your mother and me to get letters like this from you?' His father shook his head and waited for a reply but William didn't know what to say. His father gave him the letter and put his glove back on. 'You should have a think before you send any more letters like this, a good long think.' He turned back to watching the hockey. 'I thought things were going well here. What's this about?'

Where does William begin? Folding the letter in half he puts it in his pocket, he tries to steady his voice.

'It's gone wrong, Dad, I'm all alone here,' was all he could think to say.

'Well it's up to you to put it right William.' His father turned back to watch the hockey players, one boy was preparing to take a shot. Still staring across the field, he said, 'I don't want any more of these letters William.'

'I've got to leave, Dad.' William searched for words, forcing himself to keep trying to get his point across. 'I've got to leave this place.' His father tutted, almost at the same time as the player struck the ball. He turned back to face William.

'Well you're not leaving now.' He shook his head. 'I've paid your school fees for the rest of the year so you're staying.'

'Dad,' said William, but his father cut him off: 'At least till the end of the year. Then we'll see what we do.' William began to cry, which had the effect of provoking his father who straightened his back and leant forward on the bench. 'For god's sake William, don't be so embarrassing.'

'Dad I have to leave, take me with you. Please,' pleaded William. He didn't know what else to say but his father raised his hand, palm outstretched.

'Now stop!' the words shot from his mouth. He didn't shout. He didn't have to. William stopped. He sat frozen to the bench as his father looked back at the field where the goalkeeper, now flat on his stomach, got to his feet and retrieved the ball from the back of the goal.

'Pull yourself together William. Don't start snivelling. You've got to confront this like a man.' William looked down at his legs, his right knee tapping a fast rhythm all by itself, he couldn't seem to control it. His father leant closer in towards him, he felt the edge of stale breath on his cheek. 'Whatever it is, this is your own making William. You've caused this. You've got yourself into this state, this is your fault. Now get yourself out of it.' Still, William looked at the ground. 'This is a life lesson,' said his father, then his tone a note or two lighter, 'now come on, walk with me back to the car.' His father stood and waved his hand to the hockey players by way of a salute. William was thankful they didn't wave back.

Unsteady, he got to his feet. His father started to walk and for a moment William felt himself rooted to the spot.

'Come on William,' said his father, jogging him into motion. 'You'll thank me for this one day.' They walked back round the field, back past the chapel and across the road to the car park.

Then William was aware of a change in his father. He saw he had friends waiting for him in a green car, laughing amongst themselves, smoke chimneying from the open passenger-side window. His father stopped and pointed. 'Look at them,' he said to William, rolling his eyes, 'how am I going to keep them in order, eh?' William had no suggestion to make. His father reached out an arm and patted him on the back. The sudden softness in the gesture unsettled William who thought to try again; was there anything he could say? But his father spoke first, and the moment was gone.

'Keep it up now William, remember, work hard, play hard.' With that, he walked to the back of the car, took off his gloves and coat, folded them up together and put them in the boot. 'And pray hard,' said his father, his voice lighter.

They stood across the car looking at each other for a last moment.

'Christ it's cold, you never forget this cold William.' His father got into the car, said something to his friends and started the engine. One of the men waved at him and William raised his hand from his pocket, lifting his returned letter up by way of reply, the wind wrapping it around his hand.

He watched the car drive down across the car park and turn onto the main road. He took a couple of steps forward. He stood alone in the cold and watched it pass the hedgerows, pass a car driving up the road towards him, watched until it was out of sight.

All week he'd waited, and then it was over. He was stood alone in the car park watching his father drive away and trying to work out what had happened.

------•------

'I suppose I was in shock,' said William, his head tilted down, looking at the pale rug. 'I was with him but I wasn't with him. I could hardly think. I could hear myself saying things to him, but it was like I wasn't really there. I was sitting there with him, him glancing up to watch the hockey players and then looking back at me. He was more interested in the hockey than me.' William stopped and looked at me. We didn't say anything. 'I think he found me humiliating. I didn't know what else to say,' said William.

'No,' I said. William leant on one arm of the chair, he rested his head on his right hand and rubbed the skin around his temple.

'I have always felt embarrassed by the memory. I just sat there, mute, on the bench. I sat there looking at the ground while he watched the hockey.' There was a long silence. William didn't lift his head from his hand, he carried on rubbing at his temple.

'I think you were in shock, like you say,' I said.

'I didn't know what to say to him.'

'It's not clear what else you could have said.'

'I can still feel the horror I felt when he took my letter out of his pocket and gave it back to me. It was like a hideous magic trick had been worked on me. I was horrified, I felt so ashamed.' We sat in silence. I became more aware of the murmur of the school traffic outside. William leant back in his chair. He gave a little half laugh and sat upright. 'For a moment I thought he might get up and go over and talk with the boys playing hockey. As soon as he saw them he lost all interest in me. I don't think he had any idea what I was going through. I remember when he looked at the hockey I raised my hand to wipe away the tears that I could feel coming. I tried to be careful but he saw me do it, he didn't like that.' William grimaced. I nodded.

William turned his chair to the window, his face an image of unhappiness.

'I felt … forgotten. Lost,' said William. 'I felt I'd been injured, like I'd been winded.' He nodded to himself, shut his eyes and drew a deep breath. 'I think I can still feel it.'

I looked at him and digested the unhappy story. I thought William put it well.

'I'd even thought I might not be having supper at the school that night,' said William to the window. He sniffed. 'The whole thing probably lasted all of twenty minutes. Twenty minutes before I had been longing for that bell to ring, for the end of lessons. I had convinced myself that he had come to take me home. I believed it even as I walked to the car park to meet him. And then there I was, alone, still there, watching him drive away, laughing with his friends. I don't suppose he gave me a second thought.' I let out a quiet sigh. William looked at me. 'I started to cry but managed to stop myself. Taught me a lesson. He certainly taught me a lesson.'

'A hell of a lesson,' I said.

William turned his face away from me and began to cry, he tried to stop himself, but then didn't. He leant forward in his chair, put his head in his hands and cried in silence. After a while he stopped. He reached, without looking, for the tissues on the table beside him, took several and wiped his eyes in rough sharp movements.

'Oh dear,' said William. I let my gaze fall towards the floor, I could feel the emotion. 'You saying that,' said William, 'I could feel myself just well up. I could feel the tears coming. A hell of a lesson. It was a hell of a lesson. You're right. It was like all those lessons from all those years, from my cot right till then. It was all a hell of a lesson.' He wiped his eyes again. 'When you said that, it went straight through me. I am sorry, I don't mean to cry like that.'

'You didn't want to let yourself cry back then,' I said.

'I wasn't allowed to cry then. I knew as soon as we shook hands, before that, as soon as we met.'

'Yes.'

'I tried to block it out,' said William, 'to cling to the thought that I had got it wrong.' William looked down at the tissues balled in his hand, he sighed. 'But I hadn't.' He took another handful of tissues. I wondered if the box might run out. I had another box by the couch that I could give him if needed. 'If it was any other boy with any other parent, I think they would have got a different response. Even if they hadn't been taken out of the school there would have been some interest.'

'They might not have been more interested in the hockey players.'

'No,' said William, colour rising in his face. He turned and leaning towards the bin, threw the tissues in. 'And I got nothing. Just a hell of a fucking lesson, sorry. I shouldn't swear.'

'It sounds right,' I said.

'I had let myself believe that I was like those other children. Of course I wasn't. I couldn't have what they had. I didn't belong with ordinary people like them. I had let myself believe he was coming to take me home.'

William was silent, the edge in his anger passed.

'And it was Friday afternoon. The evening and the weekend stretched ahead of me.' He stopped talking.

'What did you do?' I asked, after a pause. William took a deep breath, puffed out his cheeks and sighed.

'Nothing for a moment. I remember realising how cold I was. Then I walked back up the road, towards my house, hoping I wouldn't bump into anyone. Before I got to the gate I saw a cigarette butt on the verge. It was still smouldering. Without thinking twice I picked it up, hid it in my hand and walked away from the buildings. As soon as I thought I was out of sight I put it in my mouth and inhaled. Do you smoke? Have you ever been a smoker?' He didn't wait for a reply. 'Well I sucked the smoke into me. I felt the buzz of the nicotine. I pulled on it until I was smoking the filter. Then I chucked it away. The nicotine helped, I felt sick for a moment and then this huge sense of relief. Smoking, searching out fag ends became my secret preoccupation, my obsession. My own after-school activity. After that there was nothing I was interested in except for smoking. Of course it was against the rules so I had to be careful.' He gave a sudden snort. 'It seems ironic now, doesn't it? If I'd been caught smoking I might have been sent home.' We both smiled at the thought. William looked at me smiling at him. 'You smiling at me like that,' said William, 'that's making me well up again. You're treating me as someone who has value, that's not for me. I can feel myself welling up. You shouldn't be treating me like that, I don't deserve that.' He became quiet, a pensive expression on his face. 'When I get emotional here,' said William, 'if I cry here like this, when I leave I feel different for it.'

'Different?'

'Yes,' said William. 'When I well up like this with you it changes something in me. I can feel it, it goes right to the heart of me.

It doesn't last. When I get in my car I will flip. But I feel it now, here, when it happens.'

'It makes me think of your father and his friends in the car.'

'How so?' said William.

'It just came to me,' I said, regretting I'd spoken and not sure how to follow it up. William cocked his head to one side.

'Really? I don't see that myself,' said William. I nodded, chastened. 'I don't see that,' said William, staring at me. 'I think you've got that wrong.'

I felt foolish. I shouldn't have said anything.

'I think you are putting me in my place,' I said. William looked at me, considering the thought, frowning.

'I know nothing about you.'

'What do you mean?'

'You want me to keep telling you about me. It's not very equal here,' said William.

'You don't have to say anything.'

'No I don't.' We sat in silence. 'But what's the point of sitting in silence? I could do that at home. How is this meant to work? All of this telling and retelling these horrible stories, what's the point?'

'I wonder about you asking this now, whether it relates to what happened with your father, and to your emotions welling up now?' I said.

'I don't think so,' said William. 'And I don't know how this works, but I did feel myself well up. It's strange here, I talk and you don't. It's like confession. I hadn't thought of that. It's like confession. No wonder I don't want to talk to you.' William folded his arms.

'You haven't spoken about confession.'

'I don't want to talk about that,' said William.

'Right.'

'That's another thing I don't like. You say these little words. And you nod a lot. It's like we're talking but we're not. It's me that's doing all the talking. You don't say anything.'

'It's your session,' I said.

'Yes. That's why I'm telling you I don't like it.'

'I can see that.'

'Again? That's what I mean. You don't really say anything. It's annoy-ing.' I nodded. William nodded back, shook his head and turned back to the window. 'And there's nothing in here, no books, no distrac-tions,' he gestured at the pictures, 'just these pretty pictures of hills and lakes. And of course, this,' he pointed at the Van Gogh print. I nodded. 'Why the nod?' said William. 'You're always nodding.' He turned to the Van Gogh print. 'Why did you put that picture here? Answer me that.'

'Well … I thought it mirrored the room,' I said.

'Yes, you said that before. Well I don't think it should be here. It's bad taste on your part. That's what worries me about you. The only thing I know about you is that you put that picture in here.'

'What pictures do you think I should have in here?' I asked.

'I don't know, it's not my problem.' I nodded.

'I think you should stop nodding.' William stared at me. 'Tell me something about you.' We sat in silence.

'Nothing at all?' said William

'I'm thinking,' I said. William nodded.

'Tell me more,' said William, 'what are you thinking?'

'I'm thinking what to say to you,' I said.

'It sounds like hard work,' said William. I nodded. 'Am I hard work?' said William.

'I think you were having to work hard at your school,' I said.

'No. Not at all. I wasn't doing any work.'

'Not school work perhaps. But I think you were having to work very hard to keep yourself going, to look after yourself.'

'You call that work?' said William.

'Yes. Hard work, getting through on your own like that.'

'No one else saw it like that.'

'No. But that's part of what we're doing here. We're making room to rethink things.'

'Do you rethink putting that Van Gogh print on the wall?' I gave a weak smile.

'What do you think?'

'I think I want an answer,' said William, 'I think you are hard work. I think I am very close to walking out.'

'You couldn't walk out of the school,' I said. William shook his head.

'No,' he said, 'I couldn't.' He sat looking out of the window. 'And you think me having a go at you now relates to what I was telling you about my father leaving me at the school?'

'Well yes,' I said. 'I think it might. You putting me in my place, teaching me a lesson.'

Chapter 11

William is thirteen, January has a week left to run and he won't be leaving the school permanently until the middle of June. Six aeroplane flights back and forth, Ireland to England, stand between him and the final one that will take him home for the last time. He feels a degree of anxiety all the time, it is a constant distraction. Apart from moments in art classes, he can't concentrate on any of his schoolwork.

One day in a maths lesson, the teacher suddenly shouts out his name.

'Smith!' A piece of chalk whistles past William's face and splinters against the wall behind him, he hears the pieces land on the floor.

'Jeez,' a voice behind.

'Smith!' shouts the teacher. 'What have I just said?'

William, only moments ago miles away, almost jumps out of his shirt. He startles back to attention and gulps, his lips are dry. He is aware the rest of the class are looking at him. He doesn't know what to say.

'Where were you Smith?' demands the teacher. William is blank. The teacher walks down the row of desks towards him. He reaches his arms out and brings the index fingers of both hands together so they converge on a spot in the room a few feet in front of William. 'Here,' says the teacher. 'This is where you were. Here. This empty midpoint in space.'

Everyone turns to look at the invisible point, then they look at William. William doesn't like the attention, but he is aware that the teacher is indicating exactly the point his gaze had drifted to.

'Are you looking at Westah?' whispers a mocking voice in his ear. William startles again.

'Your eyes have glazed over,' says the teacher. He throws another piece of chalk at William, it hits him on the shoulder.

'Pay attention, Smith. Focus.' The teacher stands staring at him and then walks back to the blackboard.

William feels shamed by the attention. He's relieved when the teacher goes back to explaining binary numbers to the rest of the class. The boys turn back to the blackboard—William too—but he knows the teacher is right. He has no idea how long his mind had drifted to that midpoint, he knows it is happening a lot in lessons. He just can't seem to concentrate for more than a few minutes at a time. He leans forward on his desk and looks at the ones and zeros on the board. He has no idea what any of them mean.

'I would drift. I couldn't find any peace in the school,' said William. 'Except for cigarettes. I sometimes think I should be assessed, see what's really wrong with me.'

'There was something wrong,' I said. 'But I think it's to do with things that happened to you. I think you were in a state of shock. That's why you couldn't concentrate on things. That may say more about why your mind would drift.' William looked at the ground in front of him.

'I can feel myself welling up again,' said William.

It isn't just the maths classes—he can't concentrate in any of his lessons. Everything about him at the school has changed. He has fallen out of the sports teams, his academic work is bad, his grades have gone from A to D. It must be obvious that something is wrong, but apart from the maths teacher, nobody refers to it. He spends his days drifting in classrooms or hunched in the library among the atlases and old books. There is only one thing he can concentrate on: smoking after school.

After tea, during the activity hour, when he can look for cigarettes. Smoking is his release.

Tobacco becomes his obsession. Every day becomes focused on the moment he will light a cigarette, on the relief that he knows will come then. Nothing else matters. He can't buy cigarettes so he has to hunt out discarded dog-ends. During the day, he thinks about the search he will undertake later, the lanes he will walk, the places where he tends to find them. There is a sheltered bus stop a mile up from the school. He plans each walk, each search, and the more he focuses on that, the more his mind settles.

A routine develops. Straight after tea, he puts his brown tray, plate, cutlery, and mug away in the racks in the dining hall and walks up the main road and away from the school. The weather is no obstacle and the dark winter months lend him cover. In his anorak he's just a shape on a lane. He walks first to the bus stop. He has to be careful but that is part of the kick of it, and when he's searching, he finds he can adapt to challenges as they arise. Searching for cigarettes makes him feel alive.

One night there was a music teacher waiting at the bus stop. William was just approaching the shelter when the man stepped out from the dark and looked away from him and up the road, in the direction that the bus would come. William recognised the teacher by his shiny-rimmed round glasses, but he didn't think the man would recognise him and he didn't falter or break his stride. He inclined his head a little more towards the road, stuffed his hands further into his pockets and kept walking, his pace increased a notch. The music teacher shuffled his feet, looked at his watch, and nodded an anonymous hello to the shape in the anorak. From under the cover of his hood William nodded back and kept walking. Before he was one hundred yards up the road an ancient bus trundled towards him, its weak yellow headlights scooping holes in the dark. William slowed his pace as it passed him but kept walking. He heard the bus brake, slowing to a stop, listened for the sound of the engine heaving itself away again. Only then did William turn and walk back to the empty shelter.

The first thing he did was check the timetable that was pinned to the back wall. He made a note of the time the bus had come and filed the detail away. Then he looked for cigarettes. It was his lucky night—he picked up two fag ends, one a cigarette, one a roll up, and carefully put them in an envelope in his anorak pocket.

He's found a better use for envelopes than sending letters home. He thinks of the letters he could write now.

> *Dear Mum and Dad,*
> *Am out searching for cigarettes on the school road, I have found a*
> *couple of fag ends so it's not been a bad night. Please send matches.*
> *Love*
> *William*

When he's searching like this he can even make himself smile. But he does need matches. He's got the cigarettes, now he needs the matches. That is part of the search too. Find cigarettes, preferably lit, find matches, don't get caught. That more or less sums it up. There are sometimes matches to be found at the shelter so he is on the lookout for them too. The ones with red ends are best, they are sometimes chewed and left discarded on the floor. He can't spend too long at the bus stop, someone else may appear from the school and he's already been lucky tonight. He looks up and down the road. If he had matches, he would cut across the games fields via the break in the hedge opposite and walk to the woods, where he would smoke. Afterwards he would circle back round via the art buildings, but, lacking matches, he carries on up the road, still searching, his gaze fixed on the ground ten feet ahead.

When he walks, as now, when he is searching for cigarettes and away from the school and close to the relief that comes with smoking, he is a different person. He is less anxious, he feels himself to be bolder, he doesn't have the weight of shame and rejection, he has purpose. He can concentrate.

The more he focuses on the search, the more the weight of loneliness and anxiety drops away from him. Those feelings don't go away entirely but they are masked by searching and by the anticipation of the relief that will come when he lights his cigarette. During the week he only has an hour each day. The weekends offer more opportunities, but he has to use the time he has now. So he concentrates, watches the kerb ahead, and walks.

What he likes most are the evenings when he has tobacco and matches and crosses the wet hockey fields and enters the farm track. He has learnt to be careful where he treads: the track can be rutted and muddy and sometimes full of cow shit and it's better if he smells it before he treads in it. Picking his way through the track, he comes to the woods he calls Paradise Woods. There is a stream that runs through them and that's where he goes. He likes it when he can stand with his back to the trees in the dark and draw the rough smoke deep into his lungs. There is the moment of dizziness and then the relief. As he exhales the smoke he feels a peace and lightness come over him, then he stands looking at the stream. Or when there's a break in the endless misty rain, he looks up through the branches at the sky and the first evening stars. He is still alone, but the volume of his unhappiness has been turned down. He draws out every second, he smokes whatever he has found, tatty roll-ups or discarded cigarette butts, until they are burning his lips. Then he flicks the last ember through the branches, in an arc towards the stream. On very clear nights he has heard it fizz as it hits the water, he has even seen the ember die out as it drifts down the inky dark river.

Afterwards, he draws deep clear breaths to try to take the smell of the smoke away. He packs his envelope in his pocket, and starts to pick his way up through the trees, up to the farm track and back across the fields towards the glow of the school windows. As he does so he feels his relief ebb away, he can't hold on to it, can't bring it with him, he leaves his paradise behind. Coming up by the new tennis courts he starts to think about the search he will make the next night.

This is how he measures out his days, searching for cigarettes has become everything. Being outcast he doesn't have to think about falling in with anyone else. But every so often the school presents him with a task that cannot be dodged or avoided. If he is unlucky it means he won't be able to go searching. The problem then is that all of his feelings—his anxiety, loneliness, shame, and unhappiness—come back on him, the volume turned up again. Then he feels himself to be who he is: a worthless reject cast out by his family and school friends.

It is hanging over him that he will have to go to confession this week one evening after tea. No searching, no relief, and no way of getting out of it.

William enters the chapel by the nave entrance just as a red-haired boy steps into the confessional. Another boy, head down, is walking towards William. Someone is having a lesson on the organ, stumbling over a progression of arpeggios. William thinks that will be with the music teacher he saw waiting at the bus shelter. The notes build in a sequence, then break off.

William dislikes everything about being in the chapel, dislikes the lingering smell of incense and the subdued lighting, dislikes the little wooden kiosk he has to make confession in, dislikes the priests in their long black robes. He finds the place creepy.

He steps to one side to let the boy pass, then sits on a pew and slides across to the middle of the bench. The notes start to ring out from the organ again, climbing one above another. William is glad of the music, it provides a kind of cover. He doesn't want to hear what the other boy is saying in the confessional. He worries that other boys might hear him when he confesses, though he knows it's unlikely, everyone hates confession and knows to keep their distance.

He puts his elbows on his knees and his head in his hands, he looks like he's praying but really he's biting his nails and rubbing the edge of his heels together, trying to rub some of the dried mud from his scuffed black shoes. He thinks about leaving the chapel to go searching and turns to look back at the nave door. He sees another priest standing there talking to the boy who just gave his confession. William pretends to look up at the stained glass in the tall windows, then looks back to the door. There is no escape, he can't leave now.

He doesn't want to be here. What will he even confess? He shifts his feet, levering a little more of the mud off and pushes it under the pew with his heel. He wonders who is taking confession. He has noticed a new older priest not long come to the school. He thinks about searching again, he closes his eyes and pictures himself walking up to the bus stop, being in the woods, anything to take his mind away from feeling unhappy and anxious. It works for a moment but not for long. A sequence of arpeggios breaks off again, he opens his eyes, looks back at the confessional booth and is caught again in glum sensations.

He regrets coming in, regrets everything. If he was out searching he could get away from this, but there is no way out of it now. And it's a dry night. He wonders if he might have time to walk up to the bus shelter after his confession. He looks at his watch, he wishes the boy in front of him would hurry up and finish so he can get it over with. How can it be taking so long? He doesn't need this, he just needs a cigarette, he feels on edge, a slight panic feeling, all of his thoughts and ideas are speeding up, becoming unbalanced and irregular like the organ music. When he is out concentrating on searching for cigarettes, all of these kinds of miserable anxious feelings are blocked out, all of the nervous energy dissipates. At that moment, a movement of the curtain catches his eye and derails the train of his thoughts. He looks across to see the confessional booth open and the red-haired boy step out.

William, somewhat furtive, casts a backward glance over his shoulder and watches the boy until he has left the chapel. Then he stands and walks forwards, steps in, through the purple curtain and kneels to face the grate.

'Bless me father for I have sinned, it has been one month since my last confession.'

'One month?' the priest repeats it back to him. William doesn't recognise the voice. 'And what sins do you have to confess?'

William dreads this moment, he is never sure what to say. He has to say something to get it over with, he tries to master the anxiety and unease, tries to find words. He feels himself on a precipice. The priest starts to murmur kind words to him. Somehow the kindness unsettles William, emotions shift and well up, he feels unsteady. He tries to speak but fears he might cry, he fights his tears back, then forces himself to say something. He confesses to anything he can think of, not doing his schoolwork, swearing, smoking. The priest continues to murmur kind sounds back to him through the dark wooden grate. He murmurs in Latin to William. William hears the kindness in the priests' tone, hears the voice tell him that his sins are forgiven. He tells him to make penance through prayers. He tells William he can leave. It is over.

William, lightheaded, opens his eyes wide, tries to still his breathing. He gets to his feet and steps back through the curtain to find the priest standing looking at him. It is the new priest. The priest smiles, his head leaning to one side, his mouth a gentle smiling curve, showing kind and patient eyes to William. He holds out a black robed arm and beckons William to come with him. Very surprised, William feels his emotions stir again, he knows his tears are close. He hasn't seen this coming, he doesn't want this, he doesn't want kindness, he doesn't want to weep in front of this kind old man. He tries to concentrate on other things: searching for cigarettes, the bus shelter, the things he can usually rely on to keep himself together. But now he cannot hold any of his thoughts steady.

The priest puts an arm around him and leads him to some chairs. They sit. The priest encourages him to speak. William says nothing and looks down at his shoes. The priest puts his hand on William's shoulder and squeezes. The priest spreads his hand, open, palm facing up in front of William, and tells William to put his hand on his. A few moments pass, then slow and cautious, William does as he's told. The priest puts his other hand on top of William's. The priest squeezes both of his hands together on William's, like a sandwich, then he releases his hands. William doesn't like the sudden intimacy of it and is glad to have his hand back. The priest puts his hand on William's back.

'All that tension,' says the priest, moving his hand and rubbing William's shoulder. 'And smoking? It's a bad habit. It's against the school rules too. But it relaxes you, I can imagine that.' William listens, bent over on the chair, feeling the priest's hand on his shoulder, not lifting his eyes from his scuffed and muddy shoes. The priest leans into him, he says, 'Look at me and I'll let you into a secret.' William turns to face him. The man is old, he has big yellow teeth. 'I'm a smoker myself. There, you see, now we're in it together.' The priest sits back in his chair, smiling. They sit in silence, William starts to breathe more evenly, he notices the incense smell again. He realises the organ music has stopped. 'You seem a bit more relaxed now I think,' says the priest. 'That's what confession does for you. Maybe it's me rubbing your shoulders too. Ah, maybe it's this lovely place.' The priest stops talking and they sit in silence together, the hand massaging William in slow pulses. 'No more smoking now. It's a bad habit and you'll get in trouble when you are caught. Come back to confession. You feel better, I can see that. I think you like that. Am I right? Do you like that? I think you like that.' William isn't sure what to say. He knows his emotions have calmed, he wonders if that means he likes it.

'I wasn't sure what to say. I told him I liked it,' said William. 'He was right, in a way, I did feel better.'

'I don't think you have mentioned the priest. I know you have made a link between here and confession,' I said.

'I'll tell you another link then,' said William, leaning forward and pointing, 'that purple lining of your jacket is the same colour as the sash the priests wore.' I looked down at the lining of my sleeve, feeling caught off guard.

'Sometimes I see that lining when you move your arm. I don't like it.' I felt a twinge of conscience; self-conscious, I drew my sleeves into my lap.

'It's ok,' said William, 'that priest was kind to me. Meeting him changed things.'

'How so?'

'He was good to me. I was a complete loner. Wandering around picking up discarded cigarette ends. He was good to me.'

'But you don't like to be reminded of the colour of his sash.'

'I'm not having you say anything against that priest,' said William. 'I'd stand by him in court.'

'How did we get to court?'

Chapter 12

The next night they sit together in the chapel again. They are the only people there, and there are no music lessons tonight. William wonders if the music teacher is at the bus stop yet. As before, the priest massages William's shoulders, then he moves his hands to the top of William's arms. Out of the corner of his eye William sees sparse hairs on the man's knuckles, for a moment he thinks of spiders crawling across him. William wonders when he can leave, he still might have time to get to the bus stop. The priest draws a long deep breath. William begins to realise that he won't be going anywhere tonight. He finds the silence uncomfortable, and the man's hands too, but the thing that worries him most is the kindness, William hadn't expected kindness. When he concentrates on searching, his emotions are all kept in their place. He hadn't expected the priest's kindness, and he is aware that he doesn't want it, he tries to concentrate on all the things he doesn't like.

'There's peace in here, William,' says the priest, 'and the lovely smell of the place, I feel folded into a warm blanket, do you feel that?' He looks at William's face. 'You look so unhappy William. I could hear your unhappiness as soon as you started to make your confession. I could hear it in here,' the priest taps the fingers of his left hand against his robed chest. William shuts his eyes, he can feel his emotions start to come loose from their flimsy moorings. He wishes the priest would stop, but the man is just warming to his theme. Kindness, it's the kindness that is undoing him.

'As soon as you started to speak, I thought to myself, as you told me about your sins, I thought this boy is unhappy and alone here. This boy needs a friend. Needs some peace. I'm right, aren't I William?' William is working to hold back tears. The priest seems to know it, he rubs William's shoulder. He continues: 'It's ok. I thought to myself this unhappy lonely boy needs peace and I am going to see if I can help him find that peace. Ah, that's it, let the tears come William. Those tears are angels opening up your heart.' A tear has escaped and is rolling down William's cheek. William wonders if he might just break down and cry, cry till he has washed all of the traces of mud and cow shit from his shoes. If another tear comes there'll be no holding them back. He tells himself not to cry. Inside his shoes he scrunches up his toes trying to concentrate, trying to do anything that will take his mind off this moment of kindness. He tries to still his breathing, he manages not to cry, he feels the moment of panic pass. He is trying to buy himself some time until he can leave. He tells himself it must be over soon. He wonders, if he is quick, whether he might be able to find something to smoke. He'd like to look at his watch, but doesn't think he should. He wonders, if the bus has been and gone yet. He knows that's when people tend to discard their cigarettes. But the priest appears in no mood to end the conversation. They sit together in the chapel in silence, the priest rubbing his shoulders.

'That's better,' says the priest. 'And you look like you have got some of the peace too. That's good. It's a good thing that you have come back, give us the chance to talk some more. It's good that you tell me how you are, don't worry about that. You don't need to be walking around on your own with all this unhappiness. You know what, William?' The priest pauses. William looks up at him. 'I'm going to keep this time for you, this is your time. Ok William?' His brow furrowed, wiry eyebrows raised, eyes keen, he stares at William as he waits for an answer.

'Yes father,' William responds.

'Good, good boy,' says the priest, releasing William's shoulder, his hands disappearing into the black folds of his robe. The priest stands and motions William to stand too. 'Now the prep bell will be ringing soon. You better get back to your house now, I don't want you getting in trouble. That's the last thing we want. You just come back tomorrow and we'll keep talking.'

With that William is free to leave, glad it's over; covert, he checks his watch as he walks back up the nave. There is no time for searching. He feels his irritation flare, there is no time now. If he has to return tomorrow he will have to be quick and get to the bus stop first. He could miss tea, but he's done that before and knows how hungry he was in the night. He weighs the position up, he will just have to be quick. With that, he hears the shrill peal of the prep bell ring out. Without hurrying, he traces his way round the walls of the chapel, going the long way round to delay being back in his house. He looks up at the Blessed Mary's gown, wonders about the priest. He wishes he'd had his tobacco. It's not just the nicotine he's missed, it's the freedom, the comfort of his obsessional evening searches.

When he wakes the next morning his first thoughts are about the priest, he tries to stop them by thinking about cigarettes.

Throughout the day he plans everything out. He will be first into tea and first out. He will bring his anorak with him to afternoon lessons, and after tea he will go straight up to the bus stop. He will make time, luck permitting, for smoking before meeting the priest again. He can't remember when he last had such focus. His mind is so alert that he almost understands binary maths. Even some of the teachers notice he has his concentration back. He is efficiency itself. And he is lucky. Though he is noticeably breathless when he steps into the confessional.

'That's a different type of incense altogether,' says the priest from across the partition, a trace of irony in his voice. 'You've been out smoking again.' William hears the priest take a loud deep breath. 'This is not going to do you any good William. There'll be trouble for you when this comes to light. For you *will* get caught. Then things will be very bad. I won't be able to help you then.' William kneels before the grill, penitent. He doesn't know what to say. He feels an edge of anger in the priest's words, he blows his breath towards the floor thinking he should have taken some toothpaste with him.

'Have you been out searching for your cigarettes again? Yes? Right after tea? Where do you get your cigarettes from? Do you have cigarettes on you now? Do you bring them with you from home?' The questions come one after another.

'I found a cigarette end on the road.' William says it in a rush, there is no time for making things up. A brief silence, then:

'A fag end? In the gutter?' the priest's voice jumps, his tone is incredulous.

'Yes father.' The priest is silent, then his measured words: 'This is very bad William. Are you out picking up cigarette ends, like, like a vagabond? A boy from our school?' They are both silent.

The next time the priest speaks, his voice is soft again, his words not much more than an intoned whisper from the other side of the booth. Even at that volume the kindness reaches into him. William thinks the priest's mouth must be right against the grill, he thinks of the big yellow teeth on the other side. William flexes his legs on the cushion he is kneeling on, searching for comfort.

'But I know it's only because your unhappy,' says the priest. 'You're not a bad boy, you are just unhappy and alone. And, if I say it, a bit lost too.' The priest takes a deep breath. 'Well I am glad you have come to talk to me about it, and God's glad too. Come now, let's have a chat about this in the chapel.'

William stands and pushing the curtain to one side emerges from the booth. The priest comes round to him. The building appears empty but for them.

'Come,' says the priest, putting his black robed arm on William's shoulder and guiding him towards the chairs. 'Let's sit here for a while.' They sit. 'You're not a bad boy William, I can see that. You know that don't you, William?' William, looking at the traces of mud on his shoes, nods, he notices how frayed his laces are. 'You're not a bad boy. But you are unhappy. I can see that. I can feel it in the tension in your shoulders. It's a good thing you've come to tell me about all this. It's a much better thing than carrying it all on your own. Better than walking the lanes picking up discarded cigarettes, getting all that mud on your shoes.' William fidgets, crosses then uncrosses his feet, tucks them further underneath him. The priest strokes the top of his head.

The priest's tone is kind again, like before. William doesn't want his kindness, he wants tobacco; as the priest talks William feels his emotions start to shake loose. The relief, the shield he had felt the cigarette put around him less than an half an hour ago, starts to dissolve. He feels too close to his unhappiness again. To all the things that have gone wrong. He remembers falling out with his friends, remembers sitting on the bench when his father gave him back his letter. Remembers standing in the car park when his father drove away. He remembers the feeling of rejection. The priest is right, he is alone. Talking with the priest has brought it all back to him. He feels the priest's fingers massage the top of his neck, below the hood of his anorak. He leans his head further forward, trying to pull away but not managing to. The priest tells him he is pleased with the chance to help him. The fingers knead into him, then stroke his curled blonde hair.

'I can see you like that. You know, William, I think you have been sent to me, so I can work for you.' William feels guilty for involving the priest in his problems.

'I'm sorry father.' The priest tells him he mustn't worry about anything. He tells William again that he knew the minute he saw him, that this was a boy in need of his help.

'I want you to feel better William, and that's what God wants. Look at His beautiful chapel.'

William lifts his head, he still doesn't like the place, he looks back at his feet.

'And I think maybe you do look a bit better,' says the priest, 'but I am worried about you out on the road alone looking for cigarettes. Roads are dangerous. I have a better idea. It might be,' he breaks off searching for a word, 'a little eccentric, but I think we should try it. Come and meet me tomorrow straight after tea, don't go off up the lanes, come straight to me. Ok? Ok William?' William, his mood sinking, nods. 'Good, very good. You're a good boy William, you're just a bit lost at the moment, that's all.' William, awkward, doesn't quite know what he is. 'It's good to see you looking better now. It's good that you came to me.'

All the next day William is annoyed with himself. He regrets the conversations with the priest, regrets telling him about the dog-end. He wants to stick to his routine and go searching, but his secret is out. He is annoyed with himself for talking about it. He isn't sure what to do.

He drifts through lessons, through lunch, through afternoon classes and then through tea. He leaves the dining hall and stands in the bitter cold evening, he looks up the lane. That option seems closed to him now. Then, feeling there might be trouble in letting the priest down, he walks to the chapel. The priest is waiting for him inside the main door. He smiles at William as they meet. William thinks it's all a bit of a puzzle, but he can see the priest's concern. William cannot remember when he was shown such concern.

The priest looks around the chapel, they are the only two people there, he turns to William.

'So here it is, my idea,' he says 'it will be a secret, between us. I am smoker myself. Pipe, not your horrid cigarettes. I think you should come up to my room with me now and I will let you have a smoke of my tobacco.' William cannot believe what he's hearing. There is a brief silence between them, William hears the sound of the bus trundling along the road. 'What do you say to that?' The priest looks at him, almost impish now. William doesn't know what to say. He feels a bit anxious and excited at the same time. He repeats the priest's suggestion to himself.

'Surprised, eh?' said the priest. 'Well … I said I wanted to help you, and I meant every word of it. And you won't get caught, no one will bother you in my room. None of those horrid cigarette ends you've been smoking either. And you'll be warm too. It's a cosy room.' William stands before him, speechless.

'Do you think we should do that?' asks William, not sure if it is the right thing to say.

'I have all the risks covered,' the priest replies. 'I am going to help you William. Now, shall we go? That tobacco of mine won't smoke itself.' Still William hesitates, he wonders if he has been caught up in some sort of strange prank. But he wants to smoke too, and that impulse, combined with the priest's assertiveness, wins the argument. 'Come on, I can see you want your smoke and I am going to give it to you.' With that the priest puts his arm on William's shoulder and guides him out through the side door of the chapel.

Together they walk to part of the school William has never been to, to the side door beside the school block that leads up to the priest's quarters. The area is strictly off-limits to the boys but the priest leads him now with great confidence. William, behind him, feels uneasy, unable to think how many rules he is breaking.

He follows the priest, hanging a few steps back. At the door the man produces a key from a pocket in his robe. The door seems to stick for a moment, then the priest gives it a quick shove and it yields. Turning back to William, the priest smiles, and, head tilted, waves an arm to usher him in.

Now inside, William waits, his anxiety rising, as the priest delays and looks in his pigeon hole. He stands back saying, 'Ah, it can all wait till later. But you can't, eh?' and with that the priest walks down the short corridor and starts to climb the stairs. It's almost as dark on the stairs as it was outside, the place has a musty airless smell about it and it's not very warm or well lit. William follows, keeping a few steps behind, watching the black robes sway in front of him; he doesn't like the black robes.

The staircase is mean, pinched and narrow, there are some pictures on the wall, priests together, priests in robes; he glances at them, then looks ahead. William's mind flits from one thought to another. What is he doing? He shouldn't be here, he feels a sense of guilt that he doesn't feel when he is out searching on his own. He feels the guilt compress him, he is tense, he thinks to say something to stop this now, but what? He doesn't say anything—that opportunity seems to have passed him in the hallway. Obedient, if uncertain, he follows the priest up the stairs, past gold-framed pictures of the Virgin Mary, past pictures of a gothic castle set in wide lawns. He wonders if other boys come to these rooms, he's never heard of it, but he's hardly one to know what other boys do. And if the boys knew he was there, what would they make of it? He thinks of this priest who is prepared to break rules for him, the things he is doing to help him. He hopes he won't get this kind friendly old man into trouble. He feels ashamed for thinking the priest has big yellow teeth and spiders on his fingers. He is being shown friendship and kindness, and he is going to have a smoke, and that's the thing, that's why he is here. He thinks of the relief that is to come. Tobacco: he concentrates his mind on smoking, just like when he is out searching at the bus stop. He concentrates on tobacco and tries to push all other thoughts aside. Now two floors up, it is at least warmer.

The priest's room is at the end of a corridor on the second floor. After opening the door the priest reaches into the darkness for a toggle light switch and steps inside. William waits outside, hearing the priest moving around within. The click of another light being turned on, then another, then the sound of curtains being shut.

'Come in William, don't be shy, welcome to my home,' says the priest, smiling at William, who still stands hesitating on the threshold. The priest reaches out an arm.

'Here, let me have your anorak, come in.' William notices himself shrug off his anorak and hand it to the priest. The door shuts behind him and the priest turns off the overhead light and hangs the anorak on the door, next to the priest's purple sash. 'I think that's more cosy, don't you?' William, uncertain of what to think, nods, too anxious to speak. His eyes flit from one thing to another.

Lit by the glow from a green-glass-shaded desk light and a lamp by the bedside table, the room possibly has a certain subdued cosiness about it. It's sparsely furnished. A bed, with a corner window beside it and small bedside table, a desk, and a wooden swivel chair positioned between two windows, a bookcase, a wash basin, tired hard-worn carpet, all bathed in dim light and a slight acrid smell.

'I remember thinking how black it all was,' said William. 'His robes were black, his thick leather belt was black. His rosary was black, the Bible on his desk had a black cover. I just stood there frozen to the spot. He said I should sit on the bed.'

'What did you do?'

William shrugged.

'I did what I was told. I sat on the bed, on his old tartan blanket.'

'It doesn't sound like you wanted to be there,' I said. William scratched his chin, a look of frustration on his face. I felt tension in the conversation again. We were silent for a few moments.

'I know I wanted tobacco,' said William. 'That's why I was there. But I felt guilty about it.'

'Yes.'

'This man was taking a big risk for me. He didn't have to do this. I mean, when I was out smoking the risk was all mine, but this was different. Just being up in his room was against the rules. He stood to get in trouble. Here he was taking the risk for me.'

'The way you describe it, it sounds like you were in a state of shock. I think you may have been at risk too.'

'No, I don't think so.'

'I think the way you recall the room, being stuck to the spot. It sounds like it was unexpected and strange.'

'Well there were risks, like I say. Risk is stressful. But you have to understand how alone I was. I had no one. My family had turned their back on me, I had no friends. This man was being kind to me. He was doing this for me.'

'Yes, I see that,' I said.

———————•———————

The priest sat on the swivel chair; as he moved, his heavy black robes moved with him.

'So what about this then? Up in my room, can you believe it?' he broke off and grinned. William tried to lift a smile but couldn't. 'Well I'm not sure if I can,' said the priest. 'But don't worry, you're safe here. And you look better, more relaxed. William sat on the edge of the bed, mute, unsure of himself. He didn't think he should be in the room, he didn't feel relaxed. He thinks of the tobacco to come.

'Take off your shoes,' said the priest, 'I don't want any of your smoker's mud on my nice carpet. Just relax, I'll get my pipe.' The priest turned in his chair, opened a drawer in the desk and took out his pipe and a tin containing tobacco. He turned back to William, showing him the goods. 'No, no, undo the laces, don't push them off like that, take care of your things.' He opened the tin and held it up to his nose, breathing in. William reached down and started to undo the knotted laces on his remaining shoe. 'Ahh, black cherry pipe tobacco, that's what I've got for you,' he waved the tin towards William. 'None of your dirty fag ends from the road. This is the stuff. Mind you, if you don't like it that'll be no bad thing either, might get you off the smoking all together. Ha!' the priest gave out a laugh, 'it's a win–win William, you don't get many of those in life.' William wasn't sure what that meant.

Taking his time the priest filled the pipe bowl. Next he produced a box of matches and tore a match down the side of the box. It rasped, flaring into flame, William recognised it as one of the red matches, a whole box of them. Now the priest lit the pipe and the room filled with clouds of smoke. When he was confident he had it lit he handed it to William. William looked at it, held the stem lightly, then putting it to his lips, inhaled. 'No, don't inhale, just try to savour the taste of the cherry,' said the priest.

William inhaled, he felt light-headed, felt it in his stomach and bowels too. He carried on smoking. The priest watched, smiling at William. William handed the pipe back, the priest looked at the bowl and then placed the pipe down on an ashtray.

'Your first pipe,' he said. 'Will that put you off your smoking?' William shrugged, he looked down at his grey socks. 'Well you look better,' said the priest. 'You look a lot better and I am pleased to see that.'

William tried to weigh it up, he felt some relief from the tobacco, and he hasn't had to go searching the lanes and the bus stop. He hasn't had to keep out of everybody's way, and it's warm in the room. Maybe he does feel better. But he also knows that he wants to leave now. He wished he was by himself in the woods.

'I am glad I have been able to help you,' said the priest. 'It makes me feel good to give you what you want.' They sit in silence for a few moments, William notices a ticking clock, he glances in the direction of the noise, sees the alarm clock on a shelf on the priest's dark wood bedside table. 'I like the peace, the moment after a smoke. You know?' said the priest. William did. 'You can come back tomorrow if you'd like to. Do you want to go now? Will you be okay to leave on your own?' asks the priest, his tone kind as before.

William nods, reaches for his shoes.

'Come on then,' said the priest. He stood and unhooked William's anorak from the door, careful as he untangled an arm from the purple sash, and then waited, smiling, patient, while William laced up his scuffed shoes.

Showing William out of his room he said again, 'I am pleased I've been here to help you William, you're not alone now. You have got me.' William mumbled a thank you and walked down the corridor, down the narrow stairs, past the other priests' doors, anxious that someone might come out from one of the rooms and catch him there. He felt an urgency, he didn't want anyone to stop him now. He went back down past the pictures, not sparing them a glance, his heart racing as he near-trotted to the front door, reached for the handle and pulled. It stuck for a moment and alarmed him, but then he had it open and he was outside, free. He breathed in the cold damp air.

Quick and furtive he shoved the door shut, sank his hands into his pockets, and walked away.

He walked, waiting for his heart rate to settle. He walked, drawn to the dark path that went round the edge of the main sports field, then he slowed his pace. He sat on the bench he had shared with his father a month ago. He remembered how engrossed his father had become in the hockey, remembered being given his letter back. Here he is again, feeling unsettled, relieved and guilty, his head a jumble of thoughts and feelings. He feels worried for the priest. The tobacco has left a deep, bitter aftertaste. His mouth is awash with saliva, he wonders if he might be about to be sick. Another deep breath, he calms a bit, swallows. He wishes he had a cigarette.

Despite the invitation he doesn't go back the next day; he goes out searching around the bus stop and the lanes instead. But his luck is out. As he's walking back towards his house the prep bell starts to ring. Then he regrets that he hadn't gone to the priest's room.

The next evening he goes to confession again and afterwards goes with the priest up to his room. It goes the same as before. He sits on the bed undoing his shoes. The priest asks why he hadn't come yesterday. William feels ashamed.

'Were you out searching for fag ends again William?' William nods, looking down at his socks. 'You shouldn't do that William. It worries me you doing that. I thought as much. Well I prayed that you would come back to see me tonight and here we are.' The priest leans forward, saying 'You don't have to worry about anything here William, I have got it all covered.' With that he starts to get the pipe, tobacco, and matches out from his desk. When the pipe is lit he shuffles his chair nearer to William, until William's feet are nearly touching the black robe. William leans back, trying to maintain a distance; the priest hands William the pipe.

'That's it lean back, relax, lie down if you want to. I just want you to relax when you are here. This is your sanctuary now.' William remains sitting in an uncomfortable position, leaning back, propped up on his arm on the rough green-tartan blanket, smoking the pipe. 'It's good to see the way the colour comes back to you. I can see you like it. You look a lot better, you like your tobacco don't you?' William shrugs. 'I like being able to give you what you need,' said the priest leaning back in his chair and looking at William. He tells him he will leave the front door unlocked tomorrow night—'Just come up after your tea.'

The next night William goes straight to the room.

So searching for cigarettes alone on the lanes gives way to this new activity; now throughout the day his mind is focused only on getting the priest's strong cherry tobacco.

The routine is the same with minor alterations. The priest sits nearer to William, he encourages William to lie down and smoke. William does so, it is one way to get further away from him and his big yellow teeth. The priest tells him he looks more relaxed now and that that makes the priest glad. William concentrates only on the thick cherry tobacco, the moment of relief. Nothing else matters. He is startled when the priest reaches over and touches his chest, he inhales the surprise within himself and nearly chokes. He tries to ignore the priest's touch and concentrates on holding back the cough. He starts to feel more light-headed, he blows out a stream of smoke.

'I can see you like that, touch,' says the priest, 'a bit of a massage. Well if it makes you feel better then it's good with me. Good to relieve the tension.' 'That's it,' says the priest, 'just let it all out.' William feels dizzy.

———————•———————

'I think I am going to take a break from these sessions,' said William. 'I didn't want to come today. I can't see the point if I don't want to come.'

'Do you think it might be related to what you've been talking about?' I asked.

'No. I think this may just have run its course. I've been doing this a long time. I'm not going to come forever.'

'No,' I said. 'But I think this may relate to what you've been saying about smoking in the priest's room.' William, his expression blank, looked at me, then at the knotted pine walls.

'I don't think so. I felt better when I went there, I don't feel better for talking here. Not anymore anyway. I'm sorry to say that, it's no slight on you. I just don't think this is for me.'

'I can see you got relief from the tobacco, but it sounds to me like you had become caught up in something complicated.'

'If you don't mind me saying so, I think you tend to complicate things,' said William. We both looked at each other then turned away, William looked at his right hand, I looked out of the window, thinking what to say, worried it might end here.

'I can see you liked the tobacco,' I said, 'but I don't think you entirely liked going to see the priest. It makes me think about how strange it must be coming to see me and talking about it. And I think that's coinciding now with you not wanting to come here.'

'You make everything so convoluted. And you're wrong. He gave me a lifeline. He heard what I needed and gave it to me. His room was my sanctuary.'

'Well,' I said, 'I think you were groomed.'

'What?' William jolted forward, incredulous, open-mouthed, looked at me and shook his head. 'He was giving me what I wanted.'

'That's part of how grooming works,' I said.

'He was good to me,' said William, his expression the same.

'He gave you tobacco,' I said.

William sat up, closed his mouth, then said, 'I'd defend him to the end.'

'I can see that, and this might be the end. You are talking of stopping here.'

'You think I'd stop coming here to defend him?' said William.

'I hadn't thought of it like that, but yes,' I said, 'that might be what you're doing.' William opened his eyes wide, staring at me. He considered his words carefully.

'It couldn't be that I want to stop because I have had enough of you and your ideas?'

'There's that too,' I said. 'But I think this is particular timing. I don't think you could stop going to see him, you had to go back for the tobacco.'

'You think that's grooming? You think I was groomed?' William put his keys, phone, and glasses down on the table. He sat back in his chair, looked at me, then looked away. He went to say something but stopped himself, swallowing his words. He stared into space.

'I did try to stop going, but I found it hard to go back to searching on the lanes. It was odd. Like I had forgotten how to do it. I tried to concentrate on it throughout the day like I used to. I walked around for a couple of nights searching in the bus stop and the lanes, but I didn't feel safe, it felt too risky, too exposed. I felt guilty for turning down his kindness. And all the time I was thinking I could just have gone to his room. I felt guilty, I knew he would have been waiting for me.' William stopped talking. He leant back in his chair, swivelled from left to right, then back to face me. 'When you tell me all I have to do is keep coming it reminds me of him. That's what he'd say.'

'Yes, it's complicated.'

'But I still think I need to stop. These sessions may have helped, but now I think they are making things worse. I am drinking much more. I feel terrible self-loathing in the morning,' said William.

'It's bad.'

'It's a bit worse than that,' said William.

'I think that may be to do with talking about what happened with the priest,' I said, sticking to my line. William rubbed his face. He picked up his car key and squeezed it, then he put it down.

'If we were talking about someone else, I think I might see it,' said William. 'If it was anyone else I'd feel sorry for them. Stuck there, ignored by family, unhappy, searching for fag ends. If it was anyone else, I'd feel for them. I don't know why, but I just can't feel that for myself.'

'It sounds like you're doing the opposite, taking it out on yourself, drinking more, more of the self-attacking thoughts in the mornings.'

William huffed.

'There is something in that,' he said, looking at his hands then back at me. 'You think me wanting to stop these sessions is a reaction to do with telling you about the priest?'

'Yes,' I said. William shook his head. 'And,' I said, 'I think the self-loathing you are describing, and the excessive drinking, may be part of a consequence of having been groomed.'

'Groomed,' said William, taking a deep breath. 'It's very odd how you come at things. I couldn't do your job.'

'You don't have to.'

'No, I just have to keep coming back.' William opened his eyes wide and shook his head.

———————•———————

At first, William is worried about getting the priest into trouble, he is conscious of the kindness he is being shown and is anxious about being seen by another member of staff. The curious thing is the way all of his furtive searching for cigarettes has prepared him for this; he seems able to move around the school unnoticed. Now he goes straight up through the unlocked door after tea, climbs the stairs, past the Madonnas and the faded black-and-white pictures, up to the room where he knows the priest will be waiting for him with his pipe.

He feels grateful to the priest, it scares him to think of the risks the man is taking for him. The priest makes it clear to him that he doesn't want any money or anything from William, for him it is all an act of kindness, the man is very clear about that. The massaging, like the smoking, is now part of the routine and continues each evening. William tries to ignore it. He tries to stay within himself and to concentrate only on smoking. He takes the smoke into his mouth, he always inhales it, despite what the priest says.

One evening, as he leans back on the bed, pipe in hand, the priest leans forward, pushes William's tie to one side, and starts to undo his shirt buttons. William flinches, but almost in the same moment disguises his movement, his instinct is to control his reactions. He feels the back of his shirt and vest come loose from his trouser waistband, feels the scratchy tartan blanket beneath him. He inhales, concentrating on the thick smoke and retreats with it further into himself. Next, he feels the priest put his hand under his vest and start to rub his chest. The sensation is shocking, extraordinary, there is discomfort and there is a strange pleasure in it too.

William carries on smoking as the priest continues to tell him how much better he looks. The man's hand goes lower, he starts to stroke William's stomach with light fingertips. To his dismay and embarrassment William knows he is becoming aroused. The priest's elbow brushes against the top of William's trousers, touching his erection. The priest removes his hand, straightens up in his chair. The priest seems shocked, but his expression confuses William further. Is the priest play-acting? Is William in trouble?

'Well I can see you really do like this,' said the priest. William can only think that he likes to smoke, but he feels confused and embarrassed by his erection. He hears the priest say:

'I've an idea.'

With that the priest eases his chair back, stands and goes to the wash basin, his robes swaying as he moves. From a curtain-covered shelf below the basin he picks up a white tin of talcum powder. He comes back to sit in his chair, drawing it nearer to the bed and starts to loosen William's belt and to pull down the zip on his trousers. The priest twists the top of the tin and with a puff, the palms of his hands whiten, then he reaches into William's trousers and starts to stroke his testicles.

William isn't sure if it is happening to him. He lies there trying to ignore it. He smokes the pipe, he knows he is now more involved with the priest than he understands. He feels guilt, shame, and an odd sense of pleasure.

'I know it's a relief to get what you want,' said the priest. He knows the priest is doing this because he wants him too, because it is making him feel better. He tries to fix his mind on the thick black smoke filling his chest.

William no longer prowls around looking for cigarettes. He no longer has to worry about the other boys all the time, but he does worry about being caught in the priest's room. He needn't. One day there is a noise on the stairs and an ancient priest stumbles into the room. It is just as the priest is getting the pipe ready. If he had come in a few minutes later he would have found William with his trousers and pants down around his knees. William is worried that he will be reported, but he isn't. The man makes a joke about indigestion and wind and leaves. A few minutes later the priest is reaching below the basin and getting his talcum powder out and William is lying in a cloud of cherry tobacco smoke.

So it continues, with William going up to see the priest for tobacco and the priest taking him through a slow and drawn-out routine that ends each time in him touching William. William fails to appreciate how important the routine is to the priest.

On one occasion, being desperate for the tobacco, William goes to the priest's room and without going through the drawn-out ritual, drops his trousers and pants and lays on the bed waiting to be given the pipe. The priest doesn't like it at all. William could see then how important it was to him that they go through the slow routine of it all, the careful work of the pipe being prepared and lit, the retrieving of talcum powder. The slow unbuttoning, the massaging, the stroking, all the while the priest's kind voice telling him how much better he looks. William isn't so sure. He knows he feels better for the tobacco, he also knows the days are counting down until he will leave the school for the final time. Then he'll be free.

Chapter 13

At last the summer term comes to an end. William, in his dormitory, has packed his clothes and belongings into two suitcases, one of which is still open on his narrow black iron-framed bed. With some effort he presses it shut and then carries them both down two flights of stairs to the prep room. He scans his desk, takes a last look around and leaves.

The rest of the school were at the post-prize-day tea that marked the end of the school year. William had permission to leave early, his prize was the taxi in the car park. Putting on his suit jacket and checking again that he had his passport and ticket, he heaved the suitcases up and wrestled them through the heavy black door for the last time.

He walked via the beech hedge, taking the cinder path that led round the back of the house and kept him away from the upbeat hubbub drifting from the open marquee. By the low brick wall to the side of the dining hall, where the road led down to the car park, he sat, suitcases before him, trying to contain his agitation, waiting alone until the car arrived. He was concerned in case one of the priests came over, he was also worried about missing his flight. He turned his head in the direction of the bus stop. His thoughts drifted ahead of him, he imagined the flight being delayed because of him, the passengers angry, remonstrating with the cabin staff, him being to blame for the problem. Him. How would he face them? A dusty navy Mercedes turned off the road and parked across from him, jogging him out of the problem and back to himself. A fat-faced man wearing a short-sleeve white shirt and an inscrutable expression glanced across at William. Then he looked at the two suitcases and pointed at the boot of the car with his thumb. He turned off the engine and picked up a clipboard from the empty seat beside him. William wondered if he could speak.

He put the cases in the boot, noticing as he did so a dimpled Titleist golf ball peeping out from underneath a folded chamois leather cloth; he thought of his father: what was he going to say to him now? He got into the car, sat behind the passenger seat, then watched as the driver deliberated over paperwork. William didn't want to hang around, but the driver took his time. The car smelt of stale cigarettes and cloying air freshener. The driver's ashtray was full to overflowing. William wished he had a cigarette; he thought that would be apt, him sitting in a taxi smoking while the rest of the school drank tea on the lawn. He'd have to wait.

He wound the window down an inch or two to let some of the warm July air in and then turned to look back through the rear window. The chapel, the houses, the main school block where the library was, the priest's rooms. Finally, he was getting away. He tried to hold the image of it in his mind one last time, to keep it fixed, just as it looked then, with the sunshine warming the stonework and the lawns. It looked almost inviting, like the picture in next year's brochure. Then the driver said something, and William turned back to find the man staring at him. The driver muttered again, more to himself than William and started the car. William kept looking out of the back window.

The car backed up then inched forward onto the main road, William shifted his position, twisted his neck and shoulders further and kept watching as the school receded, shrinking incrementally in his view until the buildings might have belonged in a model village, until they were gone. Only then did he turn round in his seat to face the front, noticing the driver glance at him in his mirror. William half-smiled, returning the eye contact, and then looked away, turning to let the incoming air blow across his cheek.

At the airport he bought Benson & Hedges cigarettes and smoked them one after another. He didn't have to hide now. He smoked when they called the flight, he smoked across the Irish Sea, he smoked all the way home. By the time he got back to his house his fingernails had turned yellow. This was how William went home. Home, where they couldn't ask him when he was going back to boarding school, because he wasn't. He was home for good. His father was in no mood to spend more money on his education. William was relieved to have left the experience behind him.

Part III

The coping years

Chapter 14

William, now fourteen, lived back with his family, but try as he might, he still couldn't fit in. It was the same as always, he couldn't relax, couldn't find a natural rhythm. He found he was doing things for his mother and father again, always searching, despite himself, to find the thing that would unlock the world of his family and let him back into the place where he really belonged, not this other shamed place. He felt responsible for the moods he detected in his home, he wondered if he'd brought something bad back with him from Ireland. His home was the same uncomfortable place, his mother still translating ancient Greek to herself and his father working, or at the golf club.

It was as though he were living in a different time zone, fractionally behind everyone else, a character lost in a strange story. Each night he would think that tomorrow he'd find a way to fit in, but almost from his waking moment he would have the sense that he was behind them again, that he'd missed the start. When he went downstairs he would find his mother in the kitchen already making her tea and toast and on the way to her books. He did what he could to try to catch her, but he never could.

———•———

'At least they didn't try to make me go back,' said William.

'What did you do?' I asked.

'Finished my GCSEs, then went to a local technical college, didn't do much work but I made a few friends. I was a day boy. No priests, no confession, smoke where you liked. No one taking the piss out of my accent. There was some relief in that. Not all bad. But I just couldn't settle, couldn't relax,' said William. He shrugged his shoulders, appeared to be about to say something, then didn't.

I could see he was weighed down by forces and pressures that he found difficult to name. I tried to encourage him to keep talking, keep telling me what he could and to see if we could find a way to name them together.

———————•———————

After college finished for the day he'd sometimes drink with a few of the boys he'd met. In that regard it was much easier than it had been in Ireland. They were welcoming, but William didn't follow up much on developing relationships. If anything, the friendlier they were, the more withdrawn and monosyllabic he became; he'd finish a drink with them, make an excuse, and leave.

The weeks and terms ticked by until William left school and started to look for work. He'd heard about investment companies and applied to one. He didn't get the job that he went for, but the person who interviewed him put him onto another firm that traded in metal. It was a helpful introduction and William, now nineteen, was taken on.

He was given space at a desk in a room full of people sat around trading screens. Everyone was on the phone, that's what the work involved, checking prices, offering prices. William picked things up and did well at it. He knew that his capacity to copy and emulate was behind his success, he was good at following instructions. It was noticed that he did what he was told and didn't need telling twice. His boss was pleased, the senior managers told him he'd go far; they couldn't see that William wasn't doing it for himself, that he was doing it for them, for his boss, for the managers, for the firm. They couldn't see that personal success meant nothing to him, doing it for them was what mattered to William. But they were right, he did do well, he didn't have anything else to do. Outside of work he was lost, so he worked harder, pushed himself further into the job. He stayed late at the office, stayed until the cleaners were moving about the place and locking the building up. They said if he didn't leave they were going to sweep him up with the cigarette butts. Only then would he gather his things and go. He disliked the moment when the office door fell shut behind him; other people might feel free, he felt lost.

When he wasn't working he could feel the anxiety he'd felt at school pressing in on him, it was uncanny. He couldn't understand why he felt it now. After work he'd walk away from the office smoking cigarette after cigarette, but tobacco wasn't enough, he needed something new. He started to drink, and just like he used to obsess about cigarettes, now when it got to five o'clock, he would start to think about drinking, the pub, the off-licence, his mind fixed on alcohol. He felt that some dismal emotional quality had come with him from school, a gloominess that he couldn't shake off. Alcohol seemed to help a bit and it became his focus.

At home things were changing but he wasn't paying attention. His father got a promotion and was transferred to the States. Around him his parents started to pack up and make plans to sell the house. One day he came home from work and they'd gone. He found the house empty except for a few basics, the television and his bed. He came in with some lagers and a bag of chips and found the place deserted. His parents had arranged that he could live there for two months before the new owners moved in. They'd offered to take him with them to America but he'd declined. He had a vague sense of having discussed it, that they had given him time to find a place to live, but still, coming home to find the place empty, somehow he hadn't expected it. He wondered if he'd been drunk through one of the more important conversations, or perhaps he'd been thinking about getting drunk. Perhaps he'd been in the wrong time zone and missed it. He found it hard to know how his life worked.

He put the lagers down on the floor and searched for something to sit on, found a deck chair in the garden and set it up in the sitting room. There he sat, while the sun sank through the windows behind the television and he slumped lower in his chair watching the snooker. Drinking pushed everything out of his mind. So he drank more, sitting in his deckchair, watching television until he went to bed. That was his life now: work by day, and then go home and drink himself into his bed, always alone. Because that was another thing he knew about himself, he didn't want to drink with others, he wasn't that kind of a drinker.

Before the two months were up he found a bedsit and left with the television. He was spurred into action by the new owners who came round to measure the rooms and the windows. One evening they knocked on the door just as William was starting his second lager. He didn't answer their first knock, then he saw them through the windows, walking in the garden. It was a horrible surprise. He tried to sink into the deckchair out of sight and disappear. It was no good, they'd already seen him, he had to let them in. He could see they were perplexed by his set up, him on his own, the deck chair, the cans of lager, and they knew his name, he didn't know theirs. He found a place of his own by the end of the week.

For a while he tried going to the pub after work but it never felt right. He'd feel too awkward. He'd go in, have one with some of the people he'd met, but straight away he would have an overpowering urge to be on his own. Making his way home he would be careful to go to different off-licences, the last thing he wanted was people becoming familiar with him. He started to get off his bus two or three stops early to find and visit shops that were inconvenient and further out of his way. He would try to ghost his way through the streets as though he wasn't really there.

He recognised that he got pleasure from the first drink, a lift from the alcohol, that first light rush. That moment when he'd glug the cider or lager down, drink as much of it as he could in one go and then come up for air and a huge breath and a wipe of his lips. He liked that moment, it was like the rush he'd got from nicotine at school. Precisely then, sat on his sofa, he might have a brief moment of euphoria. In that moment as the alcohol lifted him, he'd feel he was in the right time, synchronised with the rest of the world. It would be short-lived. By the second or third can he was back in his place, spiralling back into the depths of his mood, unhappy, agitated, depressed, shamed.

———•———

'You probably don't get all this do you?' said William.

'Well, I don't know if you would expect me to.'

'No, but it's what I wanted to talk about. It was the way I was alone. Coping. I couldn't find a way into things with other people. Drinking, the secret private drinking, that's always been a big part of this.'

'Part of what's kept you in your place?' I said.

'Yes, it was complicated, it still is.' He broke off and looked around the room. 'Sometimes I think I'm coming here for you not for me. Do you get that? Do you think that's strange?' He fixed his eyes on me.

'I don't know, but I can see that's what you're thinking,' I said. William kept looking at me.

'I'm not sure what kind of an answer that is. You don't know anything do you? I am not sure if you have a clue about all this. To be honest I'm not sure what you do.' He turned away, then said to the window, 'Sorry. I shouldn't speak like that.' I wondered if William might yet turn in on himself, stop talking, leave. Between sessions I worried that William would stop coming.

'It makes me think of the risk you are taking trying to trust me,' I said. 'The risk of something going wrong here, of me abandoning you. How do you trust me to be here? What about when I go on holiday? Where will that leave you?'

'Maybe,' said William, he sounded unconvinced. 'But this is older than here, these are things that came with me from school. I couldn't have pleasure for myself like the other people in the pub did, like the people in the office did. It was the worthlessness. I couldn't have anything for myself, I couldn't relax by myself.'

'You have managed to have this, to keep coming here,' I said. William grunted.

'You're always saying things like that. The thing I would say about coming to see you is the way my system sneers at it. Says I can come here for as long as I like, but that therapy will never do anything to help me. Actually, the system will be happy for me to come here for decades just as long as no progress is ever made. It would suit my system to say that you will go on holiday and abandon me, and then I will just be back in my worthless shitty place. I can't turn the system off. Ever.'

'I have thought that your system might protect you too.'

'Protect me?'

'I think the system has also kept you alive.'

'What? By keeping me in my place?'

'I think it has also kept you going. Been something you could rely on when everyone else, possibly including me, abandons you without warning.' William shook his head.

'I have spent my life trying to work out this system, what was wrong with me, how to turn it off. You're trying to tell me it's working for me? Is that what you're saying?'

'I can see you are trying to find a way to change this,' I said, trying to stick to my point. 'But I also think that this system has been reliable and kept you going too.'

'Really? That's your best yet. I should keep a book of your sayings. Kept me going? And there's me thinking it was trying to kill me all along. Fancy that.'

'I think the idea that you could work it out, do something right, gave you some hope, the hope that you could make everything better.'

William leant back in his chair. I wondered if his mood was hardening or thawing.

'You make me wonder though,' said William. 'I quite like that. I like it when you come out with something like that. I'm not sure what you're trying to say, and it doesn't make any sense when you say it, but then I feel something. Some reaction is set off, my mood lifts. But the thing is'—he leant forward, noticed I'd glanced at the clock—'I know when I leave I won't be able to hold onto the feeling.' He paused there, looked out of the window, then back to me.

'It's time to stop, isn't it?'

'Yes,' I said. William gathered his things and left.

Chapter 15

William had a soft spot for sports cars but thought of them as belonging to other people. When he needed to, he drove around London in a tired brown Austin Maxi that his brother sold to him. Sometimes when he drove the Maxi he thought of the cars he would like to drive, and one Saturday afternoon, while waiting at the traffic lights at the Hangar Lane roundabout on the North Circular he found himself admiring the MG Roadster in front of him and he had a sudden thought to buy himself one. He was twenty, he could afford it. Very unusually, the thought wasn't met with a critical onslaught laying out reasons why he couldn't, and buoyed up, as much by the thought of the car as the break in his mood, he waited for the lights to change and drove home.

He started looking through *Classic Cars* magazine until he found an MG and arranged to see it. It was perfect, finished in racing green, immaculate throughout, lovely chrome bumpers and wire spoke wheels. His offer accepted, he went to arrange finance through his bank, Barclays. Then his luck changed.

Overlooking the fact that the insurance on the Maxi had lapsed, and reckoning that it was only a couple of days until he picked up the MG, he took a chance and drove his old car to a garage in Vauxhall that had offered him a few hundred quid for it. On the way through Chelsea,

115

an elderly woman pulled out of Eaton Terrace without looking to her right. William slammed on his brakes but went straight into her. She was shaken but otherwise fine, her car was a bit damaged, the Maxi took the worst of it. A taxi stopped to help, the police were called and when they found out that William wasn't insured they threw the book at him. He ended up being given a large fine which took up most of the finance he'd arranged, and what was left paid to make the Maxi roadworthy.

William felt stupid, guilty and ashamed. He stood watching as the Maxi was towed away to the garage he had planned to sell it to, and then walked until he found an off-licence. On his table at home images of MGs stared out from *Classic Cars* magazines. He drained a can of strong lager more or less in one go. Then he collected the magazines and paperwork together and rolled them up in his hands until they formed a heavy baton. William smacked himself in the side of the head with it. Then he opened a second can. He felt it was unfair, then he turned on himself, shaking his head at his stupidity. Where had he got the idea that he deserved something nice? He slapped himself in the face with the baton again. He couldn't have a nice car. He hit himself again. That sort of thing was for other people, not him. The momentum of his anger built. By the end of the second can it was all more proof that he was a worthless piece of shit and didn't deserve anything better. He drank to that for the rest of the weekend, woke early on Monday and made his way to the office.

———•———

'Did you tell anyone what happened with the car?'

'Never. But tell me this, when I left last time I felt better. My hypervigilant system eased up, but then by the time I got home I was back in my place. Why does that happen?'

'I think sometimes something eases here, perhaps the links we make fit with that. But it's not sustained.'

'No. It's like it would be better to go off and die by myself than get help. You say that's the system working for me?'

'That makes me think of when you were winded,' I said. William stared at me, face cross, then softer.

'I thought about that too.'

'But you felt better when you left last time?'

'Yes. But the system doesn't like it. It doesn't like me feeling relaxed. It's suspicious of care.'

'I think that might be the legacy of your relationship with the priest, the suspicion might be part of that.'

'I don't think so, he gave me tobacco.' William looked out of the window. Then he reached for his wallet on the table. I wondered if he was about to get up and leave. I was aware of how involved I felt in trying to understand William's situation. Was he going to walk out now? Was this how it would end? I searched for words; what could I say if it was? That I'd failed him? That we'd failed to change William's system. William opened the wallet, he appeared to hesitate over something.

'I brought this sketch, drawing, anyway. I'm not sure if you'd want to see it. It's a sort of model.' William took a Post-it note from out of the wallet and looked at it. I hadn't seen this coming.

'I'd like to see,' I said, my interest piqued. First there was a picture of a boy in a triangle, now there was a drawing on a Post-it note. William lowered the Post-it note, raised his eyebrows and looked over his glasses at me, and puffed out his cheeks.

'Here you are then.' We stood and leant forwards to bridge the space between us, William passed the yellow square across, I sat back down and reached for my glasses.

'It probably doesn't make much sense,' said William, I lowered my glasses.

'I can see the line that divides the paper, then there's a "U", for?'

'Upper, upper tier,' said William. 'Below it there's an "L" for lower tier.'

'Right,' I said. I reset my glasses.

'I'm in the upper tier, everyone else is in the lower tier,' said William. 'Feelings, energy, libido that's all in the lower tier. You're in the lower tier too, with everyone else.'

'It's a diagram?' I said. I wondered if it might fit with the triangle image.

'It's a model of me. I'm stuck in the upper tier, in my place.'

'When did you draw it?' I said, feeling the edge of the paper stick to my fingers. William shrugged.

'Last night. I went up to my office after dinner and started sketching. I tried not to think about it too much, tried not to work things out, tried to be casual about it, tried not to set my system off. It's nothing really.'

William slumped lower in his chair, I looked at the sketch, I thought of some long-neglected element of psyche joining in with our work.

'It makes me think of a timeline,' I said. William looked up, 'a time-line running from left to right,' I said, explaining the point.

'Timeline of my life,' said William.

'Yes, perhaps. When would you date this to?'

'It's a summary for the whole lot.'

'Right. When does it start from?'

'It's the whole lot, from the beginning 'till now.'

'You used to say it started at thirteen.'

'Well, I've changed my mind on that, now it's the whole lot. Alright, maybe starting at two or eighteen months. Do you think I should put dates on the line?'

'Well, maybe'—I looked across at William—'though there's not much space on this Post-it note.' William laughed. 'Look at that, I'm laughing. We're going to need a bigger Post-it note. That's the softening again, an emotion, that's what I want more of,' he leant forward, more energised, 'To stay out of the hypervigilant system.'

'I think the softening you describe, the emotion, might be linked to the possibility of trust here.'

'Well I want more of it, but I can feel myself draw back at the same time.'

'Like the flip that puts you back in your place?'

'When I laugh I feel I break through the line, I connect with my feel-ings, my energy, I feel different anyway, but it doesn't last, that's why I want to snip the hot-wire that holds it all in place. You know, when I leave here today I'll be back in my place.'

'Above the line?'

'Yep, in the upper tier. I'm trying not to analyse this, trying to find a way of thinking about the things we speak about but without analysing them. I do see that there were traumas. That things happened to me.' He stopped there and looked at me. I looked back at him, silent and then let my gaze drift past him through the window behind. 'And the fact that you don't try to correct me, or add things, that helps me, I think it makes me feel safer with you.' I knew these were unusual things for William to say. I looked through the window, past the trees, towards the road beyond. 'I can see that things have happened to me. Well, whether

I can see it or not, I can feel that I am making connections. It's funny, but I was worried that I'd say this and that you would say something different, correct me in some way.' I was glad I hadn't tried to, I looked back at William, careful not to say anything. I knew that the slightest comment might be enough to change the whole mood. 'But then something happens here and I break through that line,' said William. 'I feel more alive. How do I keep it like that?'

———•———

By the time he was twenty-three some of William's colleagues had become concerned about him. There was nothing wrong with his work but his boss worried about the pressure William was putting himself under, all the early starts and late nights; it looked to him that William never took a break and he didn't want him burning out. He called William into his office. William stepped back from his chair. He thought he was about to be fired.

'How are you getting on William?' asked his boss. 'I mean, are you getting a break from work at all? I know you are putting in a hell of a lot of hours here. We don't want you burning yourself out.' William wasn't sure what to say. He asked if there were problems with his work.

'No, no, nothing like that. Nothing like that,' his boss almost gasped. 'I can't think I've ever suggested that someone who works for me takes a break, but you never take a break. A break can be good, get you away from the phones and the deals. Think about it, have a holiday, take a couple of weeks off, go away with your friends. You deserve it.'

William thanked him, said he'd think about it. He walked back to his desk, he wasn't sure whether he felt pleased or worried by the idea, he wasn't sure he deserved anything. He was just relieved he hadn't been sacked.

At first he ignored the suggestion, then he started to think that maybe he should take a break, if only to make his boss feel better. Should he just stay at home for a couple of weeks? No, he knew he'd just drink more if he did that. He wondered if a holiday might give him the chance to sort things out. Maybe if he took himself away he'd find a way to break his mood, a kind of reset. The idea began to grow on him, he'd go away and think everything through, and if he could find a way to start again, maybe then he'd break the cycle of self-loathing.

With these thoughts, and a small suitcase, he took himself off to a Greek island for two weeks. During the build-up he thought the idea of a holiday so unusual that he began to feel a sense of optimism. He flew to Greece, to Cephalonia, and transferred across the island to Fiskardo.

Before William finished changing out of his clothes he recognised the discomfort stirring within him. He tried to avoid it, made himself focus on swimming in the sea, and thought of the beach as he moved around his small room. It was no good, it was waiting for him in the bathroom mirror, his expression sneering back at him when he washed his hands and face. He had packed it and brought it with him, of course he had. He'd let himself think he could have something different, what was he thinking of? He slumped on his pine bed; he could fill his eyes with the sunlit sea as much as he liked, it wouldn't make any difference, none of it would, he'd still be sneering at his face in the mirror in the morning. Holidays weren't for him, they were for other people. It all became clear: the other people on the coach were in a different kind of place to him, they really were on holiday, he didn't have anything in common with them.

William had avoided alcohol at Gatwick and on the flight, conscious that he needed to be sober to sort himself out. This was the time he was going to use to clear his head, find a way out of the self-loathing, work everything out, but he'd only been in Greece a couple of hours and already he was back in his place. Because he always ended up back in this place, there wasn't anywhere else. He couldn't believe his stupidity, he had only come here to make his boss feel better. He sat on his bed, his suitcase open in front of him, some shorts, and a couple of T-shirts stacked in a pile. He had been about to put them in the creaky wooden wardrobe. What was he thinking of? He couldn't believe himself.

Instead of walking down to the beach he went to the nearest bar and started to drink, there were other people around, he didn't want to drink with them. He sat in a corner, by himself. Then he left, went to the supermarket and bought Heineken lager, went back to his villa and drank alone in the small courtyard while playing with the discarded ring pulls. He drank till he passed out. When he woke he looked at himself in the mirror and flinched. Thought he could go away to Greece and sort things out? Stupid fucker, stupid worthless piece of shit. He'd made a mistake coming here.

For two weeks he woke every morning at 5.30 am, just like he would for the office, his head throbbing. He knew the solution for this and so made sure he had four cans of Heineken in his room. He woke, drank, smoked, and read self-help books. After a couple of cans his headache lifted, after a couple more he could fall back to sleep. When he woke again it would be around 9 am and he felt a bit better.

Later, William had vague memories of sitting on the beach at night alone and throwing pebbles into the sea. Another of being on the edge of a driftwood bonfire, drinking Metaxa under a spray of stars, then falling asleep to the sound of the sea and people talking nearby. Waking later he'd staggered back up through the alleys to his room. There was sand in his bed in the morning, the window open where the mosquitoes got in.

Some days he went for walks around the rocks trying to understand what was wrong with him. His mind always turned back to falling out with the group at school, the scene by the games pitch, the ambush he never saw coming, *Wiwiam fwom Westah*. Try as he might he couldn't find a way to neutralise the mood. Sitting on the rocks scratching at his bites, he wondered if there even was a solution; he couldn't see it on land or in the Aegean Sea. The only thing he knew for certain was when it was time to start drinking again. That was his unalterable compass point. He wished he'd never let himself be talked into the stupid holiday. He made a decision that he would go back to London and sink himself further into his work; that was the one thing he seemed able to do, work. He would just have to get through this. He started to tick off the days.

———•———

'I bet you don't get this when you go on holiday. Holidays are awful for me, I shut down, I can't sit by the pool, drinking, reading books. I work up in my hotel room, I can't relax. I try to put a good face on it for the family, don't want them to see it.' He looked at the couch and then back at me. 'You know sometimes I feel alright with you. Other times …,' he broke off, leaving the thought hanging.

'You're not so sure.' I said. William hesitated, seemed in conflict with himself.

'No. I don't know. It's just the frustration, nothing changes.'

I was aware that he hadn't yet shut down here.

'I think the fact that you are able to keep coming here might be different,' I said. I was thinking of the yellow Post-it note, the timeline and the boy in the triangle drawing. I wondered what had happened to them. These were periods of high jeopardy, but gradually I learnt more of the stories of William's life from when he left school to when he started coming to see me.

So his boss found William already at his desk when he arrived for work on Monday morning. People in the office said it looked like it had done him good. William agreed, it was easier to go along with the fiction than argue. Anyway, his boss was happy he was back and that was as good as it got for William. And he did well, he bent over backwards to do a good job for them.

'You should go away more often,' said his boss, William laughed and picked up the phone.

Away from work he continued to drink by himself, it remained his secret, part of the unhappy way in which he lived. While true to his own perverse logic, in public he behaved as though he didn't touch a drop. Like when he went to the office Christmas party and drank water all evening. He watched his colleagues get drunk around him while he remained sober; late in the evening he helped them get taxis. Then he went home to his bedsit and got drunk by himself.

One night he was woken by the sound of banging, it sounded like someone was trying to break into his room. He hauled himself out of a deep sleep, wondering if the noise was part of a dream, still half-dressed from when he had fallen asleep. He lurched through his room, registering he was slipping on wet flooring. The banging continued.

Pulling open his front door he found Philip, the man from the flat downstairs, standing in his pyjamas. William could see Philip was upset about something. He tried to focus, to see if there was something he could do to help. He grasped the fact that Philip was telling him that there was water trickling through the ceiling, through the light fittings. It was raining down on his bed below, it had woken him and his girlfriend up. It came to him then, the bath. William had fallen asleep while running a bath. Leaving Philip, he stumbled into the bathroom and turned off the tap, a wave of water rolling over the side as he plunged in his hand and pulled out the plug. He tried to mop up the water with towels and placate Philip who was now standing in his room, incredulous, silent while he counted the cans and bottles spread across the tabletop. William offered Philip a drink but realised it was a bad idea as soon as he heard the words leave his mouth. The next day his landlady gave him notice to quit. She told him there'd been several complaints; he felt ashamed, he didn't argue.

He found a better flat but it wasn't available for two weeks. In the meantime he had to live in a crummy bedsit further out from London. His belongings packed in the repaired Maxi, he sloped off, not daring to catch sight of himself in the rear-view mirror.

William twisted in his chair.

'Anyway, like I say, I think I should stop coming to see you, or maybe take a break for a while. I don't think I'm getting anywhere.'

'I think when you are in your upper tier it never feels like you could get anywhere.'

'No,' said William, 'never.'

'But,' I said, attempting to develop a theme, 'I think there are moments when we're talking that you find a way out of it, when you're released from it.'

'Released from it,' said William, the words appearing to have caught his attention. At this stage in our work we lived off such moments.

'But only for moments, then I'm back in my place. This was never going to help me.'

I felt the mood sink. I recognised William might be about to throw the towel in, I knew how close we'd come to endings already. The boy in the triangle, the line on the Post-it note, was it all heading to oblivion now?

'I'm not getting anywhere,' said William.

'I'm not sure that's true,' I replied, 'you've never been able to have an alternative to being alone, it's been like that since you left school, it was like it before school. But you have been able to keep coming to see me, and I think to sometimes feel less alone here. You're sharing more of your stories here, telling me what you've been through.'

William sat still, eyes shut, I closed my eyes, opened them, swivelled in my chair, angling towards the bin, I said nothing else. We sat in silence till the end, then William scowled at me and left.

———•———

I'd think about my work with William at random times. I remember one night I woke up with a start and looked at my phone. It was 1.30 am. I lay there wondering what had woken me, hoping I'd get back to sleep. My thoughts meandered, fragments of dreams, things I'd probably forget if I didn't write them down. Then I started to think about William, about something he'd said about the priest.

'I'm not having you say anything against that priest, I'd stand by him in court.'

'How did we get to court?' I said. That was it, how did we get to court? What was it about this? Defending the priest? Is this part of how grooming works? I thought of cases that had come to light, Bradford, Rochdale, a case in Oxford, the way the girls, the victims would defend the perpetrators in court. It was hard to follow the perverse paradoxes of how attachments worked in grooming cases. It was like William's system, like everything that kept him in his place. And how did the drawings fit in with it all? Even in my dreams I tried to make sense of it.

Chapter 16

William's company was bought out, a lot of staff were made redundant but he was promoted, now he was doing very well, and at the end of the year he was given a large bonus. His father advised him to use it as a deposit and he bought himself a one-bedroom flat. William wasn't sure home ownership would change much, he knew that his mood had got worse and that when the afternoons got late, between four and five o'clock, he would become more anxious, it was like a curfew was in place. Home ownership didn't change that, he still walked through streets looking for off-licences he'd not been to before, still looked at the rest of humanity and felt ashamed. He didn't belong with them. He was twenty-five. He thought he'd be better off dead.

'But how would you do it?' came a thought, quick to pick up this thread. 'You don't like blood, you're scared of heights. You're a fucking coward.' The force of it made him cringe. Later, in his new flat, he sat alone, scared, drinking.

A week later, William drove from his home to the common and tried to gas himself. He avoided entering the car park until he thought everyone had left, then, parked in the far corner, pressed up against a willow tree with a broken branch that leant down on an overflowing bin, he tried to run a makeshift pipe from his exhaust in through the car window. He had thought it through and bought a new hoover just for the longer hose it came with, but try as he might, he made a mess of connecting the hose to the rectangular exhaust pipe and sealing the window up. He either cut off the hose or let in too much air. In the end he gave up and sat in the car drinking while the engine chugged poison in through the window. It gave him a headache, but it didn't kill him.

Afterwards, when he was back at home, and after the headache had passed, he could not get the taste of the fumes out of his throat, each black taste a reminder of his failure: he couldn't even get suicide right. He decided to go to his GP. On the phone he wanted to tell the receptionist that he was scared. He didn't, but he felt a bit better when he'd made the appointment, like he'd punctured a layer of his isolation.

His doctor was an older man with limited time for emotions. William thought his father would have liked him. He put William on Sertraline. That didn't do much for him, but he kept taking it. He kept taking it while he carried more and more bottles out with the rubbish. He had learnt to compress his bin bags before he took them out, it stopped the bottles from clinking together. He didn't want to give the game away to his new neighbours.

He took a couple of days off on the pretext of working on the flat, then he went back as requested to see his doctor. The doctor asked him how he was doing. William didn't tell him about the suicide attempt, he told him he was coping.

'Coping is a good start,' said the doctor. William nodded, pleased that his doctor seemed pleased.

'I think I am always just about coping.'

'Have you ever thought about talking to anyone about things, about the drinking?'

'No,' said William, shaking his head, searching for the right words, 'you're the first person I have spoken to in a long time, about myself I mean.' He couldn't think when he'd last spoken to anyone other than at work. The doctor nodded and looked at his notes; he laid them down on his desk, put his hands together and looked at William.

'Talking can be helpful,' said the doctor. 'We have someone in the practice, a good hypnotherapist, I think you should go to see him.' He wrote out a name and a number and gave it to William, who looked at it, doubtful. It was several days before he called.

The problem may have been that he never really took to the thin-lipped man and his ideas about aversion therapy. It may have been to do with the lack of conversation. William was hoping for the chance to speak with someone.

The hypnotherapist told him he'd create a link between William's fear of heights and his drink problems.

'Right,' said William looking around the room. But try as he did, he struggled to follow the instructions and relax; he couldn't fault the place, the lighting was calming and subdued, and the atmospheric ambient music unobtrusive. William tried to do what he was told, including—though he didn't want to—uncrossing his legs.

'Uncross your legs, just relax,' said the hypnotherapist.

Throughout the session, the thin-lipped man sat in front of him, talking, his voice even, soft, somewhat sibilant. He told William to shut his eyes, to relax and breathe.

'Just breathe deeply, in and out, in and out, that's it.' He told William to relax, as if it was a given state.

'I don't really know how to relax.'

When he left, his mood was lighter, he thought perhaps he didn't feel quite so furtive; he didn't drive straight home but went for a walk instead. He sat on a wooden bench in a park and looked at the trees, at the people playing tennis and wondered if he could play tennis again. He admired the park, the smart black iron railings, the playground, the neat hedges—he felt a peace he hadn't felt in ages. As the sun began to set he walked to his car and drove back to his flat. That night he drank, but perhaps less than normal.

As agreed, he went back to see the hypnotherapist several times. The routine was the same, but William never achieved the peace he felt after that first visit. He started to feel that the thin-lipped man was losing patience with him, the hypnotherapy sessions changed, he told William he thought he might do better with CBT. William wasn't sure what he was doing wrong, he felt he had let the hypnotherapist down, that the thin-lipped man didn't want him to come back, so he stopped going. That night, leaving work, he got off his bus three stops early, walked the streets until he found an unfamiliar off-licence and ducked in through the door.

His life made no sense to him. William had money, his own home, a nicer car, all the antidepressants he could want for. He was the most successful salesperson in the team and yet he could not shake off the feeling of failure. His success at work was all based on doing things for others, not for himself. Achievement did nothing to improve his mood.

'That's because you're a piece of shit,' whispered a voice in his head when he looked in the mirror in the morning. William nodded.

Sometimes he woke, his head pounding, and called in sick. He was never sure what the antidepressants did for him, he had his own more reliable prescription. In the morning he drove to an off-licence, bought three ready-mixed gin and tonics and the paper. Then he went to his local park and sat in his car drinking and smoking. By the middle of the second can, his head began to clear. When he was done with the paper, he read self-help books, searching for the key that would free him from his self-destructiveness. He never found it. The sneery voice told him that self-help books weren't for him. When he'd finished the third gin and tonic he drove home and went back to bed. He had known himself to pass a week at a time like this.

From time to time he picked up the hypnotherapist's details and considered calling him again, but he wasn't convinced. He decided he needed a new plan, something radical. He would take himself away again, this time he would go further than Greece, and he wouldn't come back in two weeks either.

When he was twenty-seven he sold his flat, much to his father's annoyance, left his job, went as far from England as he could, somewhere he could think things through in peace and get to the bottom of the mess of himself. He travelled to New York and then slowly made his way across the States. Late in the year he checked into the Reef Motel, Rarotonga, in the Cook Islands, there he took a studio with a lagoon view.

His room had a white tiled floor, the walls a mixture of plaster and painted brick; he liked it enough, and he didn't tend to like much. He liked the sliding glass door that led onto his veranda and there he sat in a creaky cane chair, reading self-help books, drinking and trying to think everything through. Sometimes he went for walks, sometimes he wondered if he might have found his place, here at the edge of the world.

One Sunday he hired a moped and rode round the island. It was a spur of the moment thing, he'd had a few drinks in a bar and decided to go. The barman's cousin ran the local moped shop.

As the bike swayed beneath him it dawned on him that he might have drunk more than he realised, and at a misjudged bend he came off. The bike came to a stop in a ditch, he slid across the road. He was only wearing shorts, sandals, and a T-shirt. The unforgiving roads were made of impacted coral. He came away with a bad graze on his left thigh and both forearms and limped, bloody and cut, back to the rental shop. The boys there winced at the sight of him, they wanted to get a doctor for his 'Honda rash'. He accepted the plasters and bandages but no more, he waved them away and made his way back to the bar. On seeing him, the barman frowned, shut his eyes, and looked to the ceiling where a lethargic fan turned, stirring the air.

He took his beer and tried to ease himself onto the barstool but a comfortable position was beyond him, so he stood. When he put down his glass and waved for another he saw his bandaged arm wave back at him from the mirror behind the bar. He wanted to shake his reflection off. He gave himself a weak smile and turned away, he looked through the bar's open windows and out to sea.

It had come all the way across the world with him, the über mallet, smashing all of his ideas of a travel cure and self-improvement to pieces. There was nothing he could do for himself, nowhere for him. He looked back in the mirror at the other drinkers in the bar, at the postcards from happy travellers; they were the rest of humanity, he was apart. They drove mopeds for pleasure, they took care, they put flowers in their hair, they showed themselves off. William wouldn't dream of doing any of it, none of that was for him. The barman put another beer in front of him.

William raised his glass to the barman, to all the people in the mirror.

———•———

'I went to the other side of the world, I still couldn't work out what was wrong with me. I've never been able to.'

'I don't think it's so much that something is wrong with you, as that things have happened to you,' I said. William took time to pick his response.

'I like that idea, but I can't do anything with it, I can't keep it in mind. Say it again will you?' William waited. I didn't say anything. 'When you say it, it stays with me for longer.' William closed his eyes. I wasn't sure, but I said it again.

'I was saying, it's not that there is something wrong with you, it's that things have happened to you.'

'Things have happened to me,' said William, 'lots of things.' He was quiet.

'Did you ever go back to your timeline idea?' I asked. I'd waited to see what had happened to that, William opened his eyes.

'What? Mark out the dates of all the things that happened?'

'Yes.'

'No,' said William, 'I'm not allowed.'

'In the upper tier you're not allowed anything.'

'I'm allowed to beat myself up.'

'Yes.'

'And I'm allowed to drink.'

'You would have to be in the lower tier to draw your timeline.'

'That's true,' said William, he sighed, shrugged. 'I thought, when I left school, that I was leaving it all behind, that I was free. But it all came with me.'

'I think that's right, it came with you, it's come with you here. It's what we're trying to get at now.'

We looked at each other, mirroring each other's expression, silent save for the murmur of traffic.

William's eyes went blank and seemed to fix somewhere on the wall.

Alone with my thoughts, I imagined William staring into space in the maths class, lost in space.

William swivelled his chair from one side of the room to the other.

'Where are your thoughts?' I asked.

'I was looking at the knots in your wood panelling. There's so many of them. Sometimes I see things in them.'

'What do you see?'

'Sometimes images like Munch's *Scream*, sometimes a worried frog,' said William. 'There,' he pointed. 'Do you see those three knots, those are the eyes, and that line underneath,' he drew his finger sideways, 'that's the mouth.' It started to come into focus for me. 'Do you see it?'

'Yes, I think I do.'

'Today I can pick out images.'

'Could you mark that on your timeline?'

'I'd need a lot of paper if I was going to mark down details like that.'

'You could get one of those long rolls of paper like your friend had.'

'How do you remember him?' said William, 'I don't even remember telling you that.'

———————•———————

Several days passed, his headaches got worse. The sneery voice told him he was getting what he deserved. One afternoon he stood looking out to the lagoon from his veranda, he had the momentary sense of detecting something unusual, a change in the light, something at the edge of his vision, a shimmering. He wasn't sure where it was coming from, he turned to look, he couldn't see any clouds. He realised just before he blacked out that it was coming from him.

He had his first seizure there on the sun-bleached decking outside his room. His body convulsed, he bit down on his tongue and when he came round he was bruised, wet, bloody, and confused. His mouth was cut. The motel staff found him groaning, they contacted one of the expats. A friend, the closest he had come to one, an older woman, came to see him, she wanted him to go to the medical centre and called an ambulance but when it came he refused to get in and sent it away. He just wanted to sleep, he didn't want any attention.

For the next four days he only drank water, it was the longest break he'd had from alcohol in years. And he started to eat again. He could feel his strength returning. On the fifth day he left the motel and walked to the lagoon, he waded into the crystal blue water in his faded denim shirt and khaki shorts and floated on his back, the water lapping and licking at his ears. He stayed there watching as the afternoon light changed. He was aware he was feeling a bit better. His tongue was starting to heal too. He floated there, on the edge of humanity, just trying to take things in. Maybe he had been lucky? He thought he should drink to that. With care he made his way back to the motel, showered and headed off to the bar.

The regulars in the bar were delighted to see him reappear. He drank, but not like before; the seizure scared him, and more than that he was disturbed by the thought that other people might know the state he was in, that they might realise how worthless he considered himself. He felt himself drawing back from his self-destruction, in his own way looking after himself.

Out of nowhere, a letter arrived, his sister Flo telling him she was getting married, she'd like him to come to the wedding. He thought it over, unsure at first, but began to look into the weekly flight back to Los Angeles.

He wondered if the wedding might go well, be a new start, but when it happened he felt himself an outsider. Perhaps it was the same for all of them. He didn't drink, and there were questions about where he'd been, his adventures, about why he wasn't drinking. He bluffed a bit, didn't want to get drawn into anything. His father was still unhappy that he had sold his flat. They weren't so much friendly with each other as polite. He could see none of them were particularly close. He couldn't see how to fit in and spent the evening alone at a vacated table at the back of the room. Later in the evening his brother Graham, rather the worse for wear, came to speak to him, becoming emotional, going on about growing up, his unhappy memories and nightmares about home. William shut him down, he didn't want to get into any of it.

Back in England he couldn't settle, he wondered if he should go abroad again. He wasn't sure what to do. His old boss contacted him to see what he was doing, detected William might be at a loose end and tempted him with a job offer. William hesitated but then accepted. What else was he going to do? He ended up staying for the next five years. He was twenty-eight. The same rules still applied: he was safest when working for others; his days still started with a voice sneering at him, but it never sounded so loud when he was at work.

Chapter 17

The woman on reception told him she was literally run off her feet.

'Would you mind if we go through this in the bar?' And without waiting for an answer she picked his paperwork up and waved an arm. William followed, he thought it was ironic, he'd come to join the gym and was being ushered into the bar. 'You could have a drink while you do it,' she said, 'a last drink before you start your health kick. What will you have?' William delayed, then sat on a barstool.

'I'll have a cider.' He watched her pour the cider into a glass, watched as the tiny flame of his health kick ambitions were drowned out. She gave him the drink, said she'd be back to pick up the forms, and went to serve other people. William could see they were red-faced and showered, they hadn't been waylaid. A woman came and sat next to him.

'Can I buy you a drink?'

'Why not,' said William, he could see he wasn't going to make it to the gym.

'I'm Meg,' she said waving to the woman behind the bar, who gestured back, she'd be over in a minute.

'She's run off her feet,' said William, then, 'I'm William.'

'Hello William,' said Meg.

———————•———————

Meeting Meg changed everything. There was something about being with Meg that made him feel better. He'd always say that she chatted him up, but they fell in love with each other immediately. William was thirty. Meg was divorced and had two young daughters a year apart. In time, she invited him to meet her girls. They took to William. On his own he continued to drink but when he was with Meg he drank less. He loved being with her and her daughters, he loved doing things for them, helping them. She suggested he move in with them. He talked to her about the business he would set up if he left his company and set up on his own.

'I'd do it, but it's probably too risky.'

'I think you should do it, we both took risks on each other, and that seems to be working out,' said Meg. He could see that was true.

'But where would I run it from?'

'You could use the spare room,' she said. He liked the fact that no matter which way he turned, she was still by his side.

'That sounds a bold idea,' said William.

At first it was touch and go, but then his own trading business took off.

———————•———————

For the first time that he could remember, he felt life had a wholesome purpose. In time, Meg and he married and had a daughter together. When she was born he took her with them to the river in her pram. He could never have imagined life being so good. At night he sat on the stairs listening to her playing and gurgling in her cot before she went to sleep.

The girls joked, they called him Cinderguy, like the fairy-tale Cinderella.

'Because you do everything for us', they said. It made him smile. It was so apt a name it was funny. He wanted it to last forever like this, like a fairy tale where the clock stopped and the bell never struck midnight. He was still drinking but the feelings of self-loathing had receded; doing things for his family helped him keep it under control. Looking after Meg and the girls worked for him, worked for all of them, but the problems started to return as the girls became older and more independent.

He could see they didn't need him to do things for them in the same way anymore. He encouraged their independence but knew things were starting to become difficult for him again. Being the father, the husband who was there to help, gave him a kind of cover and he was losing that, he was drinking more, and drinking in secret too. By the time he was fifty, and his youngest daughter was persuading him to let her go to boarding school, his anxieties had returned.

For weeks now the critical face with its sneering voice had been waiting for him, coming into focus in the bathroom mirror in the mornings, staring back at him with contempt, telling him he was a worthless piece of shit. Now, again, when anything went wrong—if there was a power cut, if a flight was cancelled, if there was a problem with his work—the critical voice was at him, putting him down, telling him it was all his fault. He wanted to keep it to himself, he knew a swig of gin helped that, he didn't want to worry Meg, but he was beginning to feel scared. He searched for something to do to break out of the mood that was building in him. He feared it was all going to fall apart, that he might have to leave them, creep away and drink himself to death on his own.

He went for long walks with the dog to try to think it all through. He had a lovely family, his life was better than he could ever have hoped, his business was doing well, and yet here he was, walking round fields and through woods feeling the shame and worthlessness crowding his thoughts. He could see he was wearing the dog out.

One night he decided to go for a run, something different to shake the mood, he tried not to think about it too much, put on shorts and trainers and set off. He cut through the back streets and up to the main road, turned right by the petrol station and headed away from town, over the flyover and onto the quieter lanes. It was a warm evening and looping back, because he didn't want to overdo it, he realised he had a smile on his face, he felt better than he'd thought he would. He wondered if he was feeling endorphins, the sense of pleasure was remarkable, vivid even.

Coming back over the flyover he paused to look down at the traffic. That's when the über mallet got him. The critical voice cut through, sneering.

'Running? You can't go running. Good thing, exercise, that's for other people, not you.' William faltered, taken by surprise, he stopped and held onto the handrail, the ambush had come from nowhere. He looked at the cars hurtling past below, he thought of the height to the road. Memories came back to him: crying at his old trading desk at work alone in the evenings, memories of suicidal feelings. He stood looking down, his hands clenched. Time passed, perhaps a minute, perhaps two, his feet rooting in the pavement dust.

'No more endorphins,' said the voice, 'no more running.' Scared, shamed, he forced himself to turn and walk home. He couldn't go in like this, they would pick up on his mood. He must pull himself together.

Indoors, Meg asked him about the run.

'Yes, quite good, lot of cars though,' he said, his back to her as he took off his trainers in the hall.

'I'll have a shower and be down,' he said and went upstairs. He took a long time in the shower trying to calm himself. He knew he wouldn't be going running again.

Downstairs, he grabbed a cider from the fridge.

'Thirsty work, that running. Got to rehydrate,' he said, gulping it down, trying to find the alcohol lift.

He got through dinner, drank more to lift the cloud still settled on him from the flyover. He wondered if they could see it. He was on edge waiting for the sneering voice to cut in again. After dinner he took himself away to check emails, he sat in his office, the door shut, staring at the wine glass in his hand.

'There's nothing you can do,' whispered the voice, 'they don't need you anymore, you're a piece of shit.'

He thought of the traffic speeding below him on the bypass. He thought about therapy again, remembered the thin-lipped man with his ideas about vertigo and aversion therapy. He thought of all the self-help books he'd read. He thought there must be a hard-wired defect in his brain and could almost picture a wire running across his temple to the back of his neck; he'd have liked to find a neurosurgeon with the precise tool to snip it clean away. He imagined that's how ECT worked, it must break up hard-wired connections. He Googled counsellors and psychotherapists, lists of them appeared, he looked for someone some distance away. There were so many names. He picked out the profile of a man who worked in a garden room, he quite liked the thought of that, it looked private. The voice sneered at him, told him they were all charlatans, especially the ones in garden rooms.

———•———

'It sounded like for a moment you ran yourself into the lower tier,' I said.

'I did, but I was put straight back in my place,' said William turning away. He looked at the knots in the wood until he could make out the frog looking back at him. 'I like the fact that you refer to that image.'

'I think you might like the sense that you have found a way to speak about it here,' I said. 'I wondered if you have done any more with your images?'

'No, I do think about it though, my timeline, from time to time, you know I'm not allowed to do anything with it.'

'Well, I still wondered,' I said.

'When I have time on my hands, that's always been bad for me.'

———•———

When the children were young there was plenty to do looking after them, that always gave him a break, but as they were getting older he could see that soon they would leave home; that worried him—not for them, for him. He knew when they left he would be stripped of the chance to be useful. It would be just him, Meg, and the über mallet. He would have too much time on his hands, and that was always bad for him.

Could he try therapy again? He thought of his father's old golf club friends, men who mock therapy, he thought of them raising their glasses, sneering at him. He put his head in his hands.

He stared again at the list of names, found the man with the garden room, found his website, looked at it and then before the über mallet could crush him to pieces, stood, picked up his glass and walked downstairs. He had to hold it together, he was driving his youngest daughter to her new school in a few days. Her idea, not his, he would never have considered her going to boarding school but she was persuasive, and her school said it would be good for her sport; it turned out that she was very good at sport. In the end he agreed to go and look at the place and that changed everything. Most of his anxieties dissolved before he'd parked his car, he could feel the sense of appropriate care from the moment he got there. It was miles from the dungeon he'd been dumped in.

So it was, a few days later he sat looking back through the rear window of his car, watching her going on a tour of the school. They were sad to say goodbye to each other, but she was excited too and he liked that. His daughter was confident and he had confidence in her. Then he watched her walk away with the other new girls.

He sat in his car, waiting for Meg, looking back at the school. The memory came back to him then, of the day when he was driven away from his school in the back of the taxi. He remembered wishing he had a cigarette and trying to distract himself from the driver's critical expression. He thought he would leave it all behind, all the failure, unhappiness, the sneery self-critical voice. Leave it all there at his school. He opened the window a little to let the September air in. The strength of the memory, even the air blowing across his cheek felt familiar, for a moment he worried he might start crying. He sat up in his chair, fished his sunglasses from a side compartment and looked straight ahead. He concentrated on the games fields, the buildings, the sun on the stonework and the lawns.

He glanced in the rear-view mirror, saw Meg walking towards him. She opened the door and got in, looking at him and his sunglasses.

'Very cool,' she said 'but I know underneath you're a bit sad. I am too. But she's excited. I think this will go well for her.'

'Yes,' he said starting the car.

———————•———————

'That's when I knew I had to speak with someone. I'd had your number for a while, I came back from the school and rang.'

'I think you try to avoid talking about how serious this is.'

William looked at him, bit his cheek, pulled a face.

'My death wish?'

'Yes,' I said, William turned away.

'I suppose it's there, when things are bad. I'd never do anything.'

'You did before,' I said, feeling I shouldn't let the point go. I thought I saw a flicker of interest on William's face, something surfacing, then it was gone.

'It was different then, it was just me. When …' William stopped the sentence there, dragged the words back into himself and away from the finger of sunlight reaching through the canopy of leaves and into the room. Sometimes he felt emotions well up in him like tides, only to be stifled and held back. He shook his head, as if to break the hold of himself. 'When you said that I felt something. I don't know. I want to know how to change this, but I can feel myself retreat from you at the same time.'

'When you describe emotions welling up, I think things do change, as though you come out.'

'You think I should come out?' said William.

'I think it disrupts your system when you do,' I said, fending aside the mocking tone.

'Maybe. But it never lasts.'

'I think the intensity sometimes lessens.'

'Perhaps. I do everything I can to resist it. I can't change it, it's not allowed. Like I can never have a creative idea.'

'What about your timeline? And your triangle image?' I asked. 'A creative urge is part of that, it may only emerge for seconds, but I think it's been here from the start.'

'What about them?'

'They're creative ideas.' I searched for words to follow the point up, looked to see if William would say more about what happened when the mood changed. I could feel the resistance between us but despite myself, I carried on. 'They might be a way of coming out, of remembering what's happened to you. Not just in terms of the past, but of what happens when your mood changes.'

Part IV

Adaptation

Chapter 18

Seasons passed like this. The trees surrounding my room oversaw our comings and goings. Session by session the sunlight tracked a different path across the room and as he told me more of his life I tracked developments in our work together. One of which was that William had become more able to concentrate, another was the emergence of his spontaneity. Taken together, I felt our relationship was developing a more benign quality. When we've lived through traumatic events and not been able to process them, they remain within us, unprocessed, we never find ways to adapt to what we have been through.

———————•———————

'I've noticed that I can concentrate more, that's different, I've always struggled to concentrate on anything to do with me,' said William, 'but at moments like this I can flow.' He smiled, leant back in his chair. I smiled back at him. 'Usually, I'm in the grip of my system, but now I have a feeling of freedom from that. It reminded me of the legal letter I told you about ages ago. When I wrote that, I felt good. But how do I keep these feelings?'

'Writing that letter created a way out of the system,' I said. William looked out of the window, then back at me.

'Well, I could concentrate. Like now. Now I can think about things, subjects I can never normally think of as relating to me, like trauma. But when I have time to myself, when I'm alone, then I'm lost, all negative thinking, drinking. Going over it. Trying to work out what's wrong with me.'

I thought of all the examples of William being put in his place: the cot, the school, holidays, the way he was still in his place, and the clumsy remarks I could make that left him feeling despondent, anything that might be taken as a compliment. William leant back in his chair and looked past me at the knots in the pine wooden panelling.

'Being able to concentrate is one thing, having time on your hands is a different problem.'

'I spend hours trying to work things out. Thinking it through, analysing myself.'

'Trying to think it through might be part of the problem,' I said. William raised his eyes.

'That's good. Trying to think it through might be part of the problem. I hadn't thought of it like that.' William turned away from me, looked at the walls, then back to me.

'That's neat, say that again would you.'

'I'm not sure if I need to,' I said. William looked at me.

'You mean like an obsession, like OCD? Endlessly thinking it over?'

'Yes. Like an obsession.'

'Thinking about it is part of the problem, obsessing?' said William.

'It's part of a repetitive pathway, it looks like thinking will get you somewhere but it doesn't, it's a sealed system. You go into it thinking you'll find the way out, but there isn't one, like there wasn't a way out of your cot, or school. You go down the rabbit hole again.'

'Sometimes I get out of it.'

'Sometimes. When the system is disrupted, like by Stan, or the letter, or perhaps by something here, then you find yourself outside it.'

William tapped at the armrests of the chair.

'I get a break from it, yes, but then I go back down the rabbit hole. It's a downward spiral, I go round and round. Having time on my hands, when I am by myself, it's always a problem. I remember the end of the school holidays, knowing I had to go back to school. My father wouldn't discuss an alternative.'

'Your mother never got involved?'

'No, she never did. I remember standing behind the garden shed, smoking cigarette after cigarette, crossing off the days until I'd have to get back on the plane. Trying to work out what I'd done wrong. I can still feel the tension, here,' said William, his left hand tapping his chest. I thought I could feel something of it in my own chest.

'My mother was somewhere in the house, my father was probably at the golf club, my brother and sister elsewhere. I didn't understand how I fitted in, I couldn't settle. I wish someone would snip the hot-wire that links me to this obsessional system, I think this is how ECT might work, I wouldn't want that, but I can see how it might work. Shake it all up, disconnect the whole thing, change my mood for good.'

I was never comfortable with his ECT solution but I picked up the theme.

'When connections are made here, when you have a creative idea or when you talk about certain events, perhaps then it's like the hot-wire is snipped.'

'Perhaps.' William looked away, for now fed up with my suggestions, I felt the connection between us drop out.

'Can't you just tell me what's wrong with me? What am I doing wrong?'

'I am not sure you're doing anything wrong' I said, bracing myself for an argument. 'I'm not sure you were ever doing anything wrong.'

'Look, I need more than this. I can't concentrate on anything. I need more. I can do things for others, for my wife, my family, but nothing for me. I can't even think about doing things for me.'

'You might be doing therapy for you,' I said, 'recognising your thoughts might be an alternative way to snip the hot-wire. Registering them, so to speak.'

'Registering them? I spot them and snip them off? I like that thought. I'll give you that.' The quiet became more companionable again. 'I wouldn't have thought to say that I was doing therapy for me. It's odd that I can think about this now, but when I leave I'll be back in my place. I'll flip.' I thought that was part of the point I was trying to get across.

'I think the end of the sessions puts you back in your place.'

William sniffed, looked dubious. I carried on: 'I think the flip is you being put back in your place, back in the obsessional loop. It makes me think of other endings, what happened at home, the boys excluding you at school, your father leaving you on the bench. And it makes me think of things you couldn't get out of, like the situation with the priest.' I thought to stop there, let the ideas settle between us. William turned back from the window. I thought to try to put it better. 'I think endings here might provoke obsessional thinking.' William listened, weighing the words. I felt myself relax a little. The atmosphere seemed to ease again.

'Maybe there's something in all of that. But what am I supposed to do with it?'

'That's sort of what I meant, the ending interrupts you. But it is time to stop.'

'That's not very helpful,' said William.

'No,' I said.

'That's not very helpful at all,' said William as he stood, gathered his things and left. I could see that it wasn't.

Chapter 19

William sat at home, distracted; he looked across at the wood burner then back at the near empty wine glass in his hand. He wasn't interested in the television, he'd felt different since the last session. He'd spoken about one of the art projects he could never pursue. It surprised him that he said so much about it. He felt a sense of animation—that surprised him too—but it was the way the energy from the conversation was still with him now; that was very unusual—it was unusual that he would be thinking about his interests, unusual that it should last until now. Could working on a creative project be a way of disrupting the obsessional thinking? Like snipping the hot-wire, something like that?

For months he'd wanted to work on an image. He got the idea from a Patrick Hughes' reverspective picture. He liked the way Hughes' images tricked the viewer's eyes. As you moved, the image changed, bookcases rotated, garden hedges twisted. William wanted to try to make images like Hughes did, he thought he might be able to use them for a marketing idea. There was a formula for how to produce the image; it was technical and involved a lot of maths, he wasn't confident about the maths but tonight he felt able to work on it. That was a change of perspective in itself.

He sat at his desk and opened his files: there was a photograph he had taken of the woods near his home, where the valley opened up, where he used to walk the dog, where the mountain bikers rode their bikes on the bridle path. It was a place he associated with trying to think his problems through. He checked the measurements against the formula. He'd read about how Hughes did it, he knew he had to get the maths right. He became absorbed in it, he could feel himself able to concentrate and that was a big relief in itself.

After lots of careful checking and rechecking the image in Photoshop, he printed it out and he could see as he started to fold the page into the necessary shape that it had worked. The trompe l'oeil effect created a dynamic movement on the page in his hands. As he moved the image in front of him, the valley and the wood moved too, the trees moved forward and back, the leaves appeared to ripple on the branches. Looking at it, William was more than surprised, he felt rather moved. He knew that fitted with the feeling he'd had since the session. He placed the picture down on his desk and studied it.

As he looked further into the depth of the green wood he was drawn to the movements of the pine trees. Something at the far back of the image caught his attention. A darkness, a shadow? William wasn't sure what it was. Try though he did, he couldn't make the detail out. It was like something was looking back at him; it intrigued him. He looked at his original photograph and then looked back at the print. His eyes went from one to the other.

The dark shadow wasn't in the original, somehow it had crept in, some fault in his printer? Some fault with his maths? With the way he'd folded the page? Something he'd done wrong? As he puzzled over it he could feel his mood change, he started to feel uneasy, his confidence ebbing, all the life and animation draining out of him. Right there, in an unusual moment of insight, he realised it was his success that had done it. He had no business with success, success was for other people. Then the insight itself was swept away. Shame followed. What did he think he was doing? His confidence was replaced by anxiety, it was unpleasant and familiar, he felt sick looking at the picture. He shouldn't have done this. Then a thought came, so clear it might have been whispered in his ear.

'What do you think you're doing?' It took him by surprise, it was as though someone had crept up behind him and he knew he'd crossed a line. 'This kind of thing isn't for you.' There was more threat in it now.

William felt his heart start to race, the edge of panic. Immediately, he wanted to get away from the image, he looked around his office, anywhere would do. His eyes fell on the cupboard under the window where he kept his VAT returns. He picked up the half-folded print and placed it underneath HMRC paperwork, straightened the papers on top, no one would look there. He shut it away and without turning off the angle-poise on his desk walked out of the room, pulling the door behind him shut. He stood at the top of the stairs holding the bannister, taking a few breaths.

He went back to the snug where Meg was watching television, his heart still racing. *Coronation Street* had finished, she was watching something else now. He felt relief just being with her. He stood behind her, feeling a touch awkward, he needed to say something.

'More wine?' he reached forward and picked up his empty glass.

'Yes please, just a smidge.' In the kitchen he drank gin straight from the bottle, poured himself a large glass of wine and took the bottle back to her.

'Thanks, that's enough. What were you doing?' asked Meg.

'Oh nothing, just some work I needed to finish.' He stood beside her, bottle in hand. 'What are you watching?'

'*Bake Off,*' she said, turning to look at him. 'Why are you being weird? Are you going to come and sit down?'

'Yes,' he said. He sat. Drank. Felt himself settle a bit.

———•———

A few days later, on a wet and windy afternoon, he finished telling me the story. William rushed the details and felt he should apologise for everything. I thought that in working on this creative project, William had accidentally both come out and then retraumatised himself.

'I think there may have been something in the success of it,' I said, 'something that set off traumatic feelings and memories, something that's difficult to think about or understand.'

'Look,' William began, 'I don't think this is going to get me anywhere.'

'I don't think that's true, I think you might be getting somewhere, it's unusual that you could work on an image.'

'I don't think this is helping.'

'I can see that things are bad, but I think your success set off a reaction.' William closed his eyes, shook his head.

'You don't know how bad.'

'No,' I said to his closed eyes. 'I don't suppose I do. But I think when you were working on the image, for a while you found a way out of the system and you could concentrate.' William lowered his head. 'The obsessive spiralling thinking is what needs to stop, not therapy.'

In the wooden knots in the walls, William picked out the bowed backs of three stooped concentration camp inmates toiling across the pine walls. He didn't think they would ever get anywhere either.

'I'm stuck,' said William. He sniffed, his eyes remained fixed on the inmates' backs. He remembered something Primo Levi had written about camp inmates who walked with a stooped gait in the laager, trying to avoid the camp commandant's attention. 'I can't work out what I am doing wrong,' he said. Then, more urgent, 'Why won't it stop? It's my first thought in the morning, when I shave. This relentless sneering at myself. I'm surprised I haven't cut my throat. Can you make it stop?'

'I think for a moment, perhaps for longer, something did change, you found a way out of it,' I said.

'But I went back.'

'Yes', I conceded, 'I think your success triggered a reaction.'

'I went back to banging my head against it.'

'You've been banging your head against this for a long time.'

William turned from the three inmates, he lifted his head, stared.

'And that's right isn't it, like I banged my head against the bars of my cot. Is it really that old?' His eyes widened, his expression softened. He thought back over the sequence of events. 'That image, it was strange, one moment I was concentrating, I was looking at something I'd done right. Then I panicked and immediately put myself back in my place again.'

There was a momentary break in the cloud and a shaft of sunlight caught William's right eye, he winced, swivelled his chair, the light fell on the wall behind him. 'Christ that sunlight's strong.'

He looked away, agitated, trying to find somewhere private to think. He looked at the couch. I knew William didn't like the couch. He held up his hand to block out the sunshine. In time the clouds moved back across the window, darkening the room. 'But,' he said 'when you said that, about the head-banging, it stopped. And it's true, when I worked on the image, for a time it stopped. All the head-banging stopped.

I followed an urge to work on a project. I could feel I was free of the system. Now too, at moments like this I feel myself come out of it, just like that.' William swung forward in his chair. 'Right now I wouldn't stop coming here. Now I want more. But I can't keep the feeling. I can't take it home with me. It's only when you say something like that that it changes.' He leant over, elbows pinned to his knees, looked squarely at me, a question forming. 'Have you ever worked with anyone as diffi-cult as me?' There was a brief silence, then he added, impatient, 'Just answer that will you? I need a plain answer.'

I could see he needed something.

'I think this is difficult,' I said, William grunted. The rain started to fall again.

'Not quite what I asked, but thank you.'

'You like to hear me say this is difficult.' William nodded.

'I do. You acknowledging it helps me. I don't know but there is some-thing in you saying it that I like.' He rubbed his forehead as he spoke. 'The head-banging stops. And I stop picking out dismal shapes in your woodwork.' I tried to follow his gaze towards the walls. 'I was looking at three camp inmates from a Primo Levi book, in the corner, there,' he pointed. 'I've lost them. No, there. They're stuck, like me.' He scanned the walls. 'Are these knots all the other people who came to see you and ended up stuck in your walls, shuffling about, prisoners who never got anywhere?' It was an intriguing thought. 'Sorry,' said William 'that sounded a bit aggressive, macabre too.'

'Intriguing, too,' I said.

'Damning, I thought,' said William. We were silent. I wondered about the idea.

'I think there was some spontaneity in that idea,' I said.

'What, you think that's progress?' said William.

I did. I thought that this spontaneity, William being free to express himself, might be a sign of a healthier creative life.

He cleared his throat with a cough. He sat still for a few moments. The silence was broken by the pinging of William's Apple watch. William apologised, explained, 'It's a reminder, it's telling me to move. I should have switched it off, left it in the car.' He fiddled around with the watch, then removed it and put it on the table beside his keys, wallet, and glasses.

'You need a version of that to remind you to stop the obsessive thinking,' I said.

William grunted, smiled.

'I'm not sure they do an app for that, perhaps there should be. This mood won't last, but it's good. It's like a moment of appropriate feeling for myself. Like a break in the weather. It changes everything, but then out of nothing a backlash is set off. When I leave I'll become aggressive with myself. I don't feel like that now, but it will happen. You remember Stan? My friend's dad?' I did. I could feel the flow of energy in William's mind again, feel it connecting us. 'When you treat me appropriately it reminds me of that time with Stan. I remember thinking then that I didn't deserve his appreciation.'

'Stan thought you did.'

'I thought he was wrong.'

'I think Stan's reaction knocked you out of the tyranny of the obsessive system.'

William thought about it. His eyes went back to the prisoners.

'Tyranny of the system,' said William 'that's rather appropriate.'

'Yes', I said, 'it might be part of what draws you to Primo Levi, the prisoners you see on the walls.'

'When I was winded,' said William, 'when I was five, I remember thinking then, no, knowing then, that it was better that I go off and die on my own than get help. That's what you're saying? It's as old as that?'

'Yes,' I said, 'in fact I think it may be older than that.'

'I've never been able to think something happened to me. I've always thought there is something wrong with me.' I nodded, outside the wind picked up again, throwing rain against the windows. One of the linen curtains stirred. 'But I can think and feel it now. When I am in this mood I can almost see it. It's appropriate, and I never have appropriate feelings about myself. It's precarious. But then out of nothing I'll be back in my place again, and all access to those other sensations and feelings is gone. My mind is like a one-way valve, something will trigger the change and I go through the valve and I can't come back. I think it happens with my work too, I blame myself when anything goes wrong. When a supplier lets me down, things that are nothing to do with me. Next thing, I'm back in my place with no idea how I got there. I've told you before, if a flight is cancelled, if Meg's car breaks down. Everything is my fault.'

'I think if I say something, if the mood breaks, when you work on an image, it's a moment when you're suddenly outside the obsessional system. The problem is how to keep hold of those moments.' Then I added, 'I don't think you should stop here, not yet.'

'I like it when you assert your ideas,' said William. 'It's like you stand up for me. It helps.' I was glad I'd said it. I nodded.

'It's not quite the same when you nod.' I smiled. William nodded. We sat in silence. William looked back at the wooden panelling, I looked at the clock and then out of the window.

'It is a downward spiral, a rabbit hole,' said William swivelling back to the walls.

There was a flapping of wings and a bird landed on the roof. I listened to it hopping about; it had come for something, I heard it fly away.

'I had a memory at the weekend of boarding school,' said William. 'After I had been kicked out of the group. How bleak it was. How much time there was to fill. There was nothing to break it up except for smoking. Being by myself all the time. It must have been obvious that something had gone wrong, one minute I was in all the sports teams, doing well academically too, and the next, nothing. I'm lost in space in a maths lesson and a teacher is throwing chalk at me. The point is, I felt this sudden sense of awe that I had survived it. I lay in the bath thinking about it, and I felt better for it. How do I avoid attacking myself?' We both sat quietly thinking that over.

'It's difficult, but in the bath you stopped. You were able to think, you found a way to reflect on it.'

'Yes,' said William.

'That's why you need your app,' I said, 'to help spot the moments you get caught up in the obsessive system and remind you to come back from them.'

'But why do I do it?'

'We can come back to that when you've stopped doing it.'

William smiled and shut his eyes. His thoughts drifted back to boarding school, he remembered being underneath the main school tower when the games master tacked notice of a tennis competition to the cork boards. He stepped back as William appeared.

'Smith, where have you been hiding? Have you come to sign up for the tournament?'

William hadn't, he wasn't sure what he was being asked, he was on his way to smoke with the priest but he didn't tell the games master that. 'Eh? Well don't worry, this is open to everyone. Let's put your name down.' William wondered how he even knew his name. The master took a pen from his pocket. 'There, Wednesday, 2pm, you'll be first up.' With that, the master looked at his watch, hooked his pen back in his inside pocket, and left. William stood in the cold night air listening to the master's heels clip against the red and black tiles. He looked at his name, conspicuous, the only name on the list. He heard the question again, 'Where have you been hiding?'

On Wednesday, having nothing else to do, he went to the tennis tournament and surprised himself by winning his first match with ease. He felt slightly embarrassed for his opponent. Afterwards, he sat on the grass outside the courts watching other matches play out. The rest of the day stretched ahead of him. His next game wasn't until Friday. Some boys milled around or sat in groups watching the games, but he was alone, awkward, ashamed. He wondered what had happened to detach him from everyone else like this. Sitting there, tearing up short blades of grass, he knew he'd become an outsider. It was hopeless. He had tried to patch things up with the other boys but they weren't interested. He hadn't got the heart to try again. With furtive movements he gathered his things—tennis racket, white V-neck jumper—and left, went back to his house. In the dormitory he sat on his iron-framed bed and changed back into his uniform, then he walked to the library, where he sat at the table by the window, his mind wandering vacantly, an atlas on his lap. He picked out remote islands in the South Pacific and wondered if things would be simpler if he lived there.

In the second round he was drawn against the boy who got him excluded from the group in the first place. William felt nervous and uncertain about playing but went anyway, he wondered if there might be a way to make friends again, but the boy hadn't come for friendship. The boy won the first game and made mocking remarks about *Wiwiam fwom Westah* as William prepared to serve.

More by chance than anything else, William's second serve skidded low and hit the boy right in the bollocks. He doubled up, cried out, dropped his racket. William was about to apologise but didn't. He won the match six-one.

———•———

'I got to the final,' said William. 'I felt I didn't deserve to be in it. It was for other people, not me.'

'How did you get on?' I asked. William pulled a face.

'I didn't turn up for it.'

'Ah.' I hadn't considered that option.

'It was the risk of success. I wasn't allowed success, I wasn't allowed to try and win the thing.'

'Perhaps that's like the success you'd had with your perspective picture,' I said.

William looked at me.

'I want to connect with the vulnerable thirteen-year-old me. Traumatised, alone at boarding school. I know it's talking with you that's helped me see that. Helped me to say that.' William broke off, an anxious expression spread across his face. He put his hand over his mouth, looked down at the floor. 'I'm welling up,' he said. He let out a brief sob and gulped in a breath. As quick as the moment had come, it was gone. I searched for something to say, some word that might hold the emotion. 'That's ok,' said William. 'In fact it's appropriate. I'm worried I'm going to contaminate you with my shame. I don't understand it either. I can see it wasn't my fault. I have these moments of being connected to myself. When I think of all the shit things, the shit Marmite sandwiches. What kind of home was I living in?' William put his hand over his eyes and bent his head. 'The tennis tournament, I felt I shouldn't play the final. I didn't deserve it. Now with you I think about it. If you'd been there I might have turned up for it.'

'If you'd had someone with you, it might have offered you a way out of the obsessional system.'

'You are saying a lot more about this as an obsessive thing,' said William. I was aware that I was.

'Over the weekend I had an idea to work on my project again, I made time for it. Then I heard Meg come home and I rushed to put it all away. Pure instinct. I'm always doing that, hiding everything. But only moments before, when I was working on it, I could feel my mind was in a different state, I don't know, neutral. That's very different for me, neutral. One moment I wasn't putting myself in my place. It was like I sort of reset myself, my feelings about myself. Of course it didn't last. I think you know it wouldn't last. In fact, I like the fact that you know. Any idea of something being for me and I'm back in my place. Like the excitement I felt about packed lunches. Anything that's for me creates anxiety, vulnerability. I turn on myself, blame myself, shut everything down. When I make an appropriate connection with you it's like that hard block of Kerrygold butter melts, no more shit sandwiches. You remember that?'

'I do.'

'Ireland. Boys taking the piss. I was reading a blog about boarding schools, the stiff-upper-lip stuff. There were stories of abuse too.' William broke off, raised his eyes, looked up at the ceiling. 'I was thinking about the way the priest touched me. I remembered when I got an erection, I was horrified, I felt my body was betraying me. The priest touched me with his elbow and then jumped back. I think he pretended to be shocked. He said he could see I really did like this. I was horrified.'

'I think he confused you, he always implied that you wanted it, but you didn't, you only wanted to smoke,' I said.

'I was horrified, and there was my erection.' He broke off. 'I don't think I was groomed.'

'I think he used your vulnerability and his tobacco. I think him jumping back, pretending to be surprised was all part of the grooming. Always making it look like you wanted something, that he was only doing what you wanted. That's how he groomed you.'

William looked at me, silent. I wasn't sure what would follow. I waited, letting my gaze shift away to the window behind William, to the trees beyond.

'I know I feel better for having talked about it. And the state I was in, the sense of feeling worthless, I can see that was there before boarding school.'

'I think that was the vulnerability the priest picked up on.'

'Maybe.'

'Grooming has made the sense of self-blame worse, the depth of the downward spirals worse,' I said. William was silent for a while. I knew he didn't like me suggesting he'd been groomed.

'I saw a programme about Savile, about how he abused people. There was a woman in the programme who said she had been abused by her grandfather when she was small. She said that she thought she had the word "vulnerable" tattooed on her forehead. That predatory people like Savile could see it. You think I was like that?'

'Yes, I think that's right,' I said, 'you were vulnerable.'

'Careful,' said William. I gave a half-smile.

'I well up when you smile at me like that,' said William. He turned back to look at the knots. 'I dreamt I went to see a psychologist, psychiatrist, someone like that. I kicked off my shoes, brown shoes, and lay on a couch. It was a sanctuary.'

'Ah,' I said. William seldom told me about his dreams.

'I thought you'd be interested in that,' said William.

'Sanctuary?' I said.

'Yes, that was the word.'

'What did you make of it?'

'What did I make of it? I don't know, I didn't make anything of it. Maybe it made me think of here. I don't know if I would have thought to call this a sanctuary.'

I felt rather encouraged by the dream. A sanctuary.

Part V

Creativity

Chapter 20

William squeezed through my door, a brand-new art portfolio folder wedged under his armpit. He put his wallet, keys, and glasses on the table, and the folder by his feet. He took off his jacket and placed it on the end of the couch. I noticed the jacket being put there; it was unusual for him to have anything to do with the couch, and it made me think of him kicking off his shoes in the dream. I was also rather interested in the folder.

'Look at that,' said William to the jacket, then to me, 'do you think I'm finally settling in? Putting my jacket on your couch.' He leant back in his chair. 'How are you?'

'I'm ok, thank you,' I replied, glancing at the jacket. 'How are you?' William nodded.

'I'm ok too, thank you.' He swivelled in his chair, looked around the room, scanned the knots and checked his bearings. 'I have been thinking about your app, my app, coming out, the timeline idea, maybe that could be a way to remember. Remember what's happened to me. Stop me going down the rabbit hole, something like that. It's been unusual, but amidst the drinking and recriminations I've come back to it and I'm not normally allowed to think like that. I've had the sense of having a visitor's pass to humanity during some of our sessions. And after them too.' He looked back at the knots, quiet for a while. 'I mustn't be flippant, I have to be careful about this. The slightest thing will put me back in my place.' I wondered where he was going with this. 'I am look-ing at you more too,' he looked at me, then turned away. 'It's like there's an impulse in me trying to make an appropriate connection with you. Sometimes when I'm driving here, I think of my father, his temper. Sometimes about being with the priest. On the wall over there, now, I see those three inmates, there in the knots in the pine, I think they're walking around a concentration camp. But when I look at you now, it seems to keep my whole self-critical system out.' He shut his eyes, shook his head.

'Anyway, I tried to draw that timeline idea, the aide-memoire, I brought some drawings, they're nothing special but I thought I'd show them to you before the über mallet gets me.'

'I'd be interested to see them,' I said, cautious not to say anything that might upset this opportunity. William looked at me, weighed the position.

'Well,' he said, 'I feel I've tried everything else.' With that he started to open the folder and took out several very large sheets of paper. He flicked through them, stopped at one, placed it on his knees. I could see a black line running horizontally from one edge of the page to the other. What looked like a curved arrow ran from the top to the bottom, another curved arrow ran back to the top, I couldn't really make the details out. It looked technical. It reminded me of the Post-it-note sketch. William was quiet, he looked at the image.

'Could I see it?' I asked. William looked up, then reached forward. We both stood. William handed me the image. I fished for my glasses then looked at the paper.

'Other way. That's the wrong way up. It's my system,' said William.

'Right' I said, turning the page.

'I am in the top, above the black line, that's the upper tier. That's my worthless place, but then I make an appropriate connection with myself, or with you, and I find a way into the lower tier. I join up with the rest of humanity. But then … you see the arrow going back up?' he pointed. I did. 'Then something happens and I'm put back in my place in the upper tier.' I kept looking at the image aware that William was watching me. 'Does it look stupid? I should probably just get back in my place and have done with it.'

I looked up.

'I don't think you should do that,' I said, delaying returning the image, concerned in case William's enthusiasm suddenly collapsed altogether. 'I don't think you should stop this. Not yet anyway.' I looked back at the image, wondering about the upper and lower tiers. 'Why did you put yourself above the line, the upper tier?'

'It's just how I saw it. You mean you'd expect above the line to be a good place?'

'Yes, perhaps,' I said.

'When everything went wrong, I think my world exploded in a trauma, I think I was thrown up there. Into the upper tier,' said William, 'that's why I'm up there.'

'Are there more images? I'd be interested to see them if there are.' I stood, reached forward and returned the image to him.

William took it back, held it in his hands. He looked for a moment like he might crush it into a ball. I waited, quiet, I thought of the über mallet, hanging above our heads.

William left the image on his lap. Then he put his hands over his eyes and started to cry. He cried, mute, then he lowered his hands and settled them on the arms of his chair; he stretched his eyes, took a few breaths.

'I feel a bit better for that. When I well up like that I feel the whole system fall away.'

'Perhaps that's what an appropriate connection feels like,' I said.

'It doesn't last, it's never sustained.'

'Maybe not, but I think a connection gets made. Is that like you being in the lower tier?' I asked, looking at the page on William's lap. William looked down at the image. He nodded.

'Yes. I could feel for myself. When I asked for help from my parents, when my father came to the school and sat me on that bench. I thought he would help me, but he did nothing, worse than nothing, he told me I deserved to be there.' His voice grew louder as he spoke.

'I think the emotion you felt just now, I think it brought you out of the grip of the obsessional system, your feelings flowed.'

'Why don't they train teachers to spot vulnerable and abused children?' William raised his voice as he spoke. 'You can't expect an abused child to speak about it. I watch these programmes about abused children, look at the charities saying they are there for children, that children can come and talk to them. It's ridiculous. Abused children can't go and talk about it. A traumatised child doesn't talk about it, they feel too ashamed to. People need to be trained to spot what's not being said, spot the behaviours.'

I thought how well William put things like this. William was silent.

'I don't know who I was before all of this happened. If I'd lived a normal life until I was twenty-five, and then something traumatic happened, then I think I would have had something to fall back on. I would know who I was before. But I don't remember who I was.'

'No,' I said.

'I think that's the difference between me and my siblings, that's why we drifted apart. They had some experience, they were either a bit older, or much younger. I can feel there is a side of me that wants to reach out and connect with you, and another side that wants me to get back in my place. It's very unusual, I can feel both things happening at the same time. Both sides of me. How do you trust someone to care for you when there has been no care, no trust?' We looked at each other, the question hanging between us. 'But after the last session, and after welling up now, I don't feel cowed or put in my place. I thought about things you've said, like the fact that I am the only trader I know who is still going. You're right about that. All of the others went bust, got divorced. And when I thought about it, I felt good,' he tapped his chest, 'actually good. Then later I thought about the timeline idea. Thought of drawing images that would help me remember what happened to me, what happens to me when I flip. Then I lost my concentration, put myself in my place and drank a bit.'

William broke off and looked at the floor. We sat in silence.

'You've come back to it though. Are there other images?'

'A couple more.'

He reached into the large folder and took out two more sheets. I watched as William seemed to wonder where to put them.

'What about if we put them on the desk?' I said, 'then we could look at them together.'

'Can we do that?' said William, uncertain.

'I don't see why not,' I said.

'I thought that would be against the rules.' I gave a half smile. We both remained in our seats, then we stood and went to the desk.

In a measured way, William put three pages down on the desk, one at a time. 'It's the timeline, they link together,' said William. 'They represent my time at boarding school, and then afterwards.'

'Right, I see. I wondered if you had done more with this.'

'I haven't really known what to do with it. This is the start, boarding school,' said William. I looked at the images.

'Have you thought of putting a panel before this one?' I said. 'Something to show what went on before you went to boarding school?' William shrugged, uncertain. I produced a lined A4 pad and removed a sheet of paper. I laid it on the left of William's images. 'You could continue your timeline back across here,' I said. 'Have you thought of putting any images on the line?'

'I'm no artist, I can't draw,' said William.

'I don't know if you need to be, maybe use any images, cut out images, maybe just words.' We didn't need a work of art.

'Like a collage? A mood board? Use emojis?' said William.

'Why not. You could use any image that would help develop it. That image you drew of the triangle. You, the boy in the triangle, maybe that could go in?'

'I haven't thought of that in a while.'

'I think drawing the timeline might be a way of remembering things that have happened to you and that might be a way of interrupting the obsessional thinking. Reconnect you to the you who wells up, the impulse to come out. It would be interesting to see what being able to keep those links in mind might do for you.' I could feel the hope in my words, I didn't mean to burden William with any of my own expectations.

William looked from one image to the next.

'I like looking at this with you. I like the fact that you are interested and suggesting things. It makes me think of my friend Paul, him unrolling paper, saying we can draw what we want. I could put dates on it, my age. I could include therapy with you, put an image of you in the lower tier looking up at me.'

'Yes', I said, I smiled, 'you could.' I wondered where he might go with this.

Later that evening, while coming back into the sitting room to refill Meg's glass, an item on the news about the planned return of the Bayeux Tapestry to the UK caught William's attention. He stopped pouring wine and lifted his head just as Meg changed channels on the television.

'Can you turn that back?' said William. He handed her the bottle and she gave him the TV remote. He was just in time to catch the end of it. He saw a familiar detail, an image of a soldier pulling an arrow from his eye, perhaps King Harold. The camera panned across other images, the newsreader commented on the consistency of the needlework. Someone from the British Museum said something but William wasn't paying attention to the words. It was the tapestry that had his attention. He gave Meg the TV control back. 'I want to check something,' he said and left the room.

Up in his office he trawled Google for images of the Bayeux Tapestry, marvelling that it was seventy metres long. He had always known about it, remembered looking at it at school but not paying much attention. Now it fascinated him.

Chapter 21

'There was a piece on the news about the Bayeux Tapestry,' said William. 'And I thought about what we've been saying here, about timelines, stories, telling my story in a series of connected pictures.'

I thought of William the Conqueror, realising I was picking up on William's enthusiasm. I thought I should watch out in case I started to sound too enthusiastic.

'And I think you're right,' said William, 'my timeline wouldn't have to be grand, I could use any images to tell my story.'

'All the things that have happened,' I said.

'You know it was all stitched by nuns? I can't get away from Catholics.'

'Perhaps an image of the priest could go on it?'

'Him?' He paused, lowered his head and looked at the knots on the walls. I felt a change in the mood. 'I'm worried I'm suddenly going to flip and lose my momentum,' said William. 'When I can keep this all in mind, I feel free of the system. Then I'm not in the upper tier, I'm somewhere else. But I can't always keep it in mind.'

'I wonder if my mentioning the priest might have disturbed you.'

'I'm not sure. Maybe. But I think last time, when you suggested we look at the images together at your desk, it had quite an effect on me.'

William swivelled in his chair, looked out of the window then back at me. 'It made me think of when my father came to the school, when he sat me on the bench, the shock of that moment, I thought he was going to rescue me, but instead he put me back in my place. I think you suggesting we could look at the images together was like the opposite of that. Instead of him producing my letter from his pocket, you offered to look at the images with me.'

I thought William made a rather good link.

At home William started to draw and work on images. He found it did help him to develop perspective on himself, his history, his moods and feelings, his rabbit holes and introspective spirals, and the act of making the images released his long-held impulse to create. He drew, collaged, and built up a picture of himself in time, his history. He found he could concentrate on it, though not always for long. There were times when his mood would drop away, his focus lost.

Sometimes he came back to me saying it was pointless. We talked about it. William talked about being back in his place, the upper tier, just like in the images he was creating, only now he could point to the spot.

'I go back to this one, panel number five, I call it the coping panel,' said William, holding up the page. I thought it rather neat that he was using his own illustrations to explain himself. When the work faltered, I was interested to know what had happened to disrupt William's concentration. I guessed that the dips in mood related to things that happened to him. Perhaps to memories and feelings stirred up by working on the images. Perhaps to other things: home things, work things or obscure things like a flight being cancelled. I tried to test out the idea that the dips in mood weren't random, they coincided with things.

'I think this is something you might have to learn how to do,' I said. 'Perhaps you have to keep exploring the idea that you can reflect on yourself, that there is more to you than the system and the upper tier.' I stopped talking, I wasn't sure where William was, or that I was putting it well. What could I say? 'You might have to keep practising it,' I said, trying again. William nodded.

'I did have a problem at work.'

'What kind of problem?'

William went back through the train of his thoughts.

'Well, in fact, one of my suppliers had a problem and it disrupted everything. They made a mistake, and it created a problem for me.' He stopped there, thinking it over. 'You think that sort of thing affects my mood?'

'Well, it coincides with your dip in mood.'

'That's fair. I wouldn't have thought of it like that, it coincides. When things like that happen, my mood flips. It might not have anything to do with me. Might be something ridiculous like a plane being late. I should include that. Maybe this could be an app.'

———————•———————

William shut the office door and looked at his desk. He was about to put the artwork there, but then thought better of it. If he did, he would have to move everything when he started work again and this might take time. The table to the side of his printer would be better. He cleared the assorted files stacked up on it and put them away on the shelves. Then his mind went blank. He sat in his swivel chair. A few minutes passed.

He pulled up images of the Bayeux Tapestry. Could he be Harold dying on the beach? Could he be William the Conqueror? Is another outcome possible? Perhaps something less heroic or defeated than either of them? He decided to run with it for the time being. It would do as a model. Because he hadn't seen that coming, Julian offering to look at the images with him at his desk in the garden room. He played the moment over in his mind. He remembered he didn't feel alarmed and that in itself was unusual; if anything he felt encouraged. He felt safe, like they were sharing an experience. They had looked at the images together, like partners. Appropriate. A sense of trust? Perhaps. He remembered feeling he was enjoying the proximity, standing side by side, and at the same time thinking to himself that he would have to go home and think about it on his own. That's what he was doing now. And the drive home had been different, no detours to off-licences, none of the sneering eyes in the mirror, no abusive flipping, no über mallet. He still had his shoes and coat on. He removed his shoes, thought of the brown shoes in the dream, sanctuary. His mind was elsewhere, back in the garden room. He bit his lip, then went over to the table and put the papers down.

He reached for an A4 pad and wrote the words 'über mallet'. An über mallet would have to be included. Yes, he would make a list of the key objects and put them in the panels.

A cot, a door slamming, a boy squashed in a triangle, cigarettes, a priest, gin, and an über mallet: those would do for starters. He put the pad down. He laid the panels out on the table, the way they had done together. For a while he just sat looking at them. 'Don't put pressure on yourself,' he said to himself, 'be easy to break this mood.' He thought he sounded like Julian. He Googled the Bayeux Tapestry again, scrolled through pictures. He looked to the Tapestry for context.

> In the Bayeux Tapestry William sits to a feast with his nobles and Bishop Odo says grace. Servants load food onto shields to carry it to the banquet.

He detected a mood of doubt spreading over him like a cloud blocking out the sun, he started to feel he might not be able to do it. Then he thought of Julian being there, looking at the images with him; that gave him a nudge.

There were the images, and there was the memory of looking at them together. He recalled the moment.

'What about if we put them on the desk?' said Julian, 'then we could look at them together.'

'Can we do that?'

'I don't see why not.'

He'd thought that wouldn't be allowed. He hadn't seen it coming. Like Stan. Like Paul with the roll of paper. Like the random moments that break up the obsessive system, that snip the hot-wire, moments when he could come out of his place.

He went back to the images of the Bayeux Tapestry, the details, he looked at the stitching. William's army rides, the English soldiers stand on foot.

'Just draw,' he said to himself and the empty room. 'Get on the beach and draw.' He nodded.' And don't start nodding.' He took up his pen and drew a timeline the way Julian suggested, the way he saw it when they were together.

He'd got stuck, not knowing where to put things when he did it before, but now he drew a timeline along the bottom of the page and started to add dates and events to it.

Far left he put a 13, far right he wrote the number 60. He was 60 years old. He looked at the numbers. He conceded there was no point starting at 13. He crossed 13 out and put a 0 in its place, told himself not to worry about the crossing out. The crossings-out would be part of the story. He noticed his adaptability. From 0 to 13, that's a story in itself, perhaps that was the main story.

He drew a line across the middle of the page; parallel with the time-line below, it divided the page into two halves, two tiers. That's how it was: him in his place in the upper tier. He didn't fit in with the rest of humanity, the rest of humanity was in the lower tier.

Did he ever fit in? That made him think. Yes. Like now, like today when he was talking with Julian, standing by the desk he felt like he did. Like he was given a guest pass to humanity. He wasn't stuck in his place on a bench with his father. That would have to go on this too.

> ... a feast is prepared in the open air, chickens on skewers,
> a stew cooked over an open fire and food from an
> outdoor oven.

There were singular moments when he felt himself tap into something different, like the moments when he welled up in the sessions. All his life he had worked to try to hold the emotions back, the impulses of himself. It went against the grain, but it was better when he didn't hold the feelings back, when he let himself feel, when he let the emotions go through him. Grief? Shock? He wondered what to call them. When he let the feelings through, he didn't feel alone or in his place. It felt appropriate.

He was aware that he was concentrating and the sensation made him smile. Being absorbed in it, not put in his place, being like this was entirely different, his breathing, his body and mind felt settled. Concentration was generally only for other people, for what his family wanted, for what his business needed. But here he was concentrating on himself. He guessed that for once he must be in the right time zone, he had caught up with himself and with everyone else. He looked at the images before him. Was the dividing line always there? No, he thought, because it wasn't there now. He thought Julian would like that observation. William put today's date on the timeline and then Tippexed the dividing line above it. Right now there was no division. William was tier-less, with the rest of humanity, like he was with Julian. It happened today in the session and he had brought it home with him and it was still going on now. He'd not been dumped back on his arse, horrified by his father on a school bench, the door slammed on him again. This was something else.

He thought about other breaks in the dividing line. Was there a time when there wasn't a line at all, when he wasn't divided? When? He couldn't think when. When he was a toddler? How small must he have been? Now there were so many images and ideas in his head, the timeline kept going wrong, or he would remember something and try and add it in, then nothing fitted right. But instead of giving up, he got more paper and started again, over and over again. He was surprised by his stamina and adaptability.

William played with the idea that once upon a time he had been different. That there might have been a time before everything went wrong, before he was put in his place and left there, before his mind became split like a page divided. Before he was emulating people and doing things for everyone else in the role of a boy named William who lived in the wrong time zone and had to make sure he was doing what other people wanted. Before he was William the Emulator.

He pushed back in his chair, straightened his legs and realised he hadn't even thought about drinking. Then he remembered that Meg would be home soon, that he hadn't done anything about supper. Should he stop? If he stopped, would he be able to start again? He didn't want to stop. He liked the feeling of concentration. He was in flow, he pressed on.

He started on a new page, it would be the first panel, it wasn't divided into two tiers. He wrote a 0 on the left corner. He drew himself as an infant playing in the garden, sitting on his mother's lap. He pictured a mug of hot chocolate, a trampoline, a football, a paddling pool, a boy flying a kite: an idyllic time in the sun, before the first catastrophe, before everything went wrong, a time before trauma. A time when he was in the right time, when everything was right. Then he drew an explosion, wrote the word 'boom!' in big letters in the middle of it, drew himself being left in his cot in the upper tier and the door slammed shut on him. That's when the dividing line began.

He marked this as him at two years old, his new starting point. This was where it all began, the first trauma. That marked the end of the

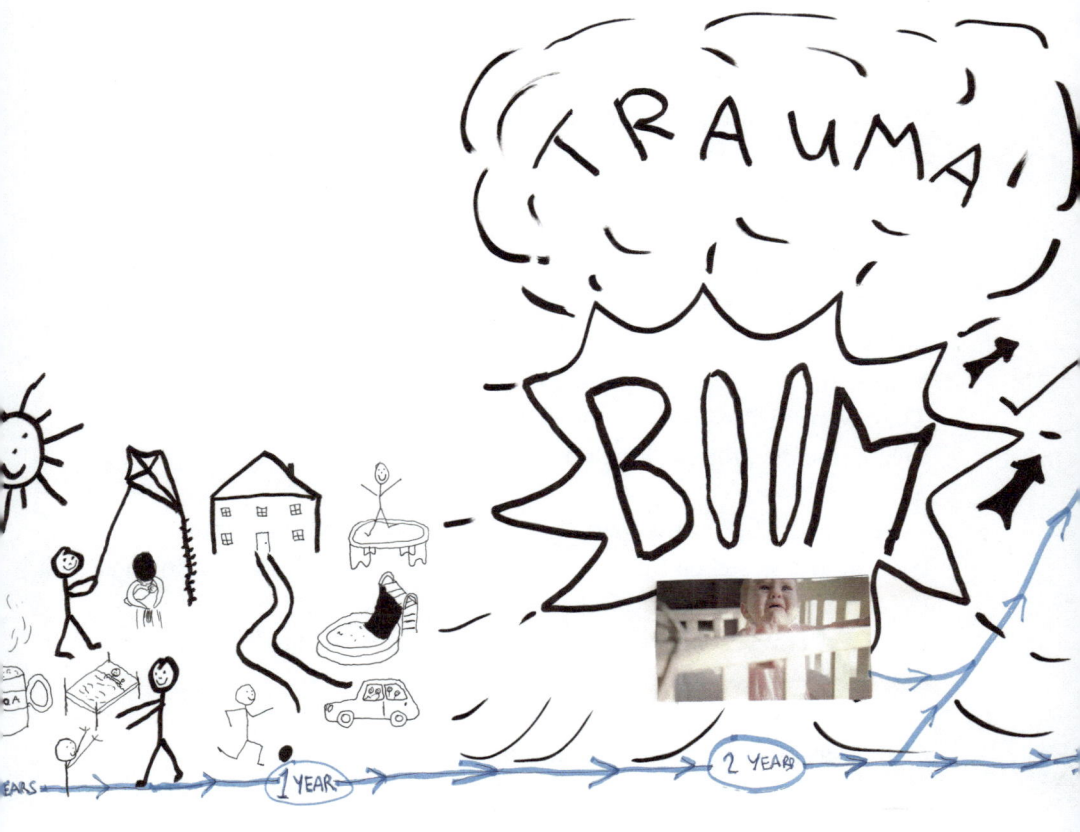

Panel 1: years 0–3

first panel, the end of the undivided him. He rubbed his hands together, the thought of it seemed to chill him. An arrow in the king's eye in the Bayeux Tapestry. He thought about cider, gin, red wine, anything to get the arrow out. Drink, it was imperative, the thought sounded like an independent voice within him, like a herald on the beach. Yes, he said to the thought, but not now. He tried to focus on the page, hold the line. He wanted to fire an arrow back in the eye of his obsessive system. On Google he found a silhouetted picture of a man drinking straight from a bottle, pouring it down his neck. He wished he could draw and paint like Paul Nash but he tried not to become self-critical—that would have been easy. He printed and cut the picture out and stuck it on the panel with a Pritt stick.

He thought about things he couldn't really remember but which he thought might be true. Like being left in his cot waiting for his mother or his father to come and rescue him, only they never did. He realised that all the waiting alone in his piss-soaked nappy, banging his head, must have changed him. The way his mother had changed, the way the relationships with Graham and Flo had changed. They were older when everything changed at home, they'd had a head start on him, in being who they were. That's why they weren't as worthless as him. Julian had talked about that. How one trauma left him changed, vulnerable, set him up for further traumas and more vulnerability. Now the ideas banged against his head. So many soldiers shouting, pouring across the beach. They were in his house. A noise downstairs, the front door shutting, Meg home, her voice calling up to him.

'Hello?'

He put the lid on the Pritt stick and placed the scissors down, leant back, stood, stretched his arms to get the stiffness out. Looked down at the images. He thought to hide it all away, but he didn't. He could show it to Meg? Not yet. He walked to the landing and called to her as he went down the stairs.

'Someone's in a good mood,' she said. He wondered if it was that obvious as he walked with her into the kitchen.

Later, after dinner, after she started watching something he didn't want to, he went back to his office. Normally he would check emails, but he didn't do that now. He went to the other table, back to the project. Panel two, in his place, in his cot. Left there. Waiting.

> In the Bayeux Tapestry William has built a castle to shore up the Norman position.

After all that waiting he was changed, divided like the horizontal line that cut the panel in two.

It wasn't just being put in his cot, it was the waiting that followed. Did waiting combine with the sense that he was to blame for what had happened? Was everything his fault?

The second panel, William from two to five years old, was awful and unrelenting. In the upper tier the images of William were grainy, and all in black and white, in the lower tier the images were in colour and the people there were happy. He used the triangular image too—him in his worthless place, the image he'd shown Julian long ago. Now, as he drew,

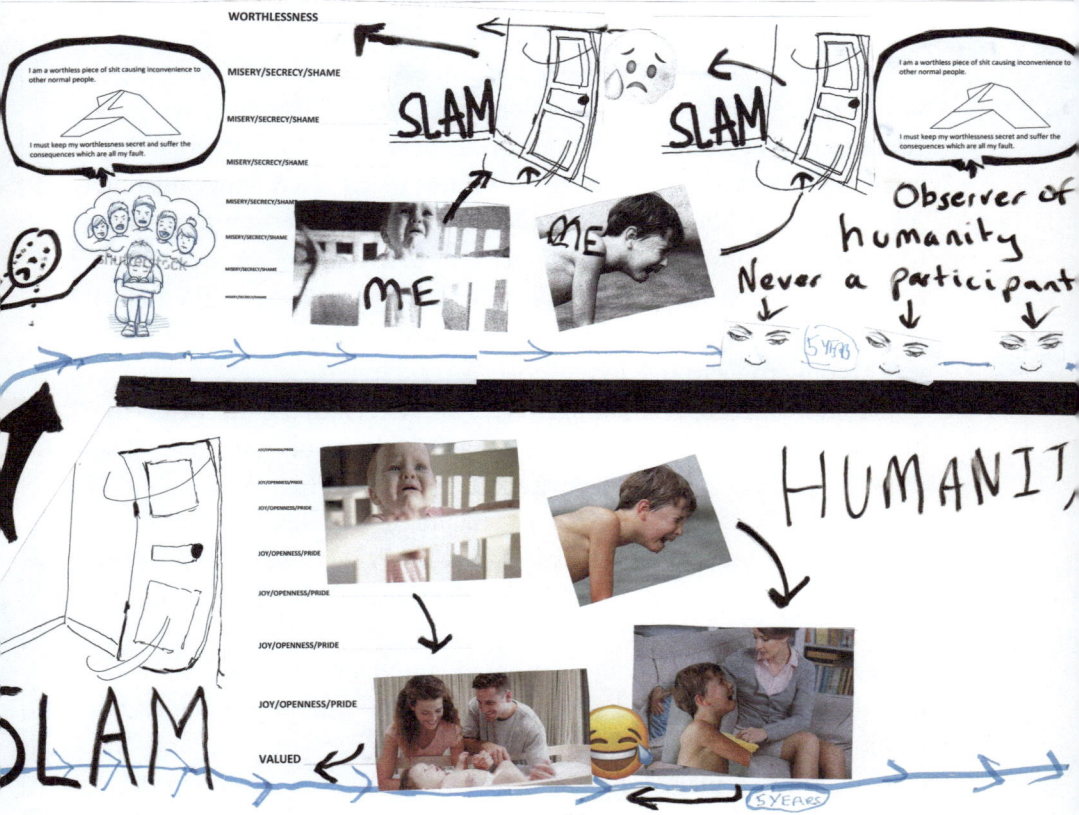

Panel 2: years 2–5

he thought of being set apart from the rest of humanity. Being in his place, his role, distraught or spending pocket money on his parents, cleaning, doing things his brother and sister didn't have to do. Doing anything he could to make things better for them.

Did the obsessional emulating all start back then? All he knew was that he wasn't himself anymore, he'd become a lost imitation of himself, endlessly worrying about what he had done wrong while he tried to catch up with the rest of them. Don't be late, emulate. That was his place. He stuck in black-and-white grainy images of unhappy children, images printed from Google, some cut out of newspapers and supplements. He put them all in the upper tier, above the line, all unhappy, all images of him. Him as a baby, toddler, infant, boy, adult. As he worked, the images became harder to manage.

Humanity was below the line in the lower tier. There, the same images were stuck, but they were in colour and clear: those children were comforted, no one slammed doors on them, they had value, when they cried they got appropriate attention. He was in his place, above the line. Amongst the pebbles and the bodies and the driftwood on the beach, worthless. An observer in the upper tier, desperate to work out what he'd done wrong, not part of humanity anymore. That was the mainspring of his obsessive ideas because emulating people in the lower tier was his only route to freedom.

He took a break, realised again that he was enjoying the work, the pleasure of being able to concentrate. Concentration, pleasure these were things he tended not to have access to. And yet here he was, enjoying this. This was what Julian had said, and he was right, doing this he was finding a way out of the obsessional loops. This was snipping the hot-wire, coming out. Stepping back from the endless spiralling thinking. And when he could do that, things changed.

Laid out like this he could see how his problems started way back, that they'd never stopped. Now when he had time on his hands, or when something went wrong in the world, everything became his responsibility. A plane being late, a terrorist attack, a world currency crisis, a tsunami, something going wrong for Meg at work, anything at all. All these things became his fault and he was put straight back in his place. Back in the upper tier, worthless, back in the cot, back in the school where his father left him. Then all he could do was things for other people. He was William the Emulator, waiting to be rescued. He became the vulnerable abandoned two-year-old version of himself.

... a messenger brings William news of Harold's army.

The memory of his father's words: 'These letters have got to stop, William. Do you have any idea what it does to your mother and me to get letters like this from you?' He remembered the horror when his father gave his letter back, it was like he could still feel the shock of it. He never saw that coming. That's how his old fears were made, how the repeated shocks and disappointments became part of his understanding of who he was. But working on the images now was disrupting the system. He found

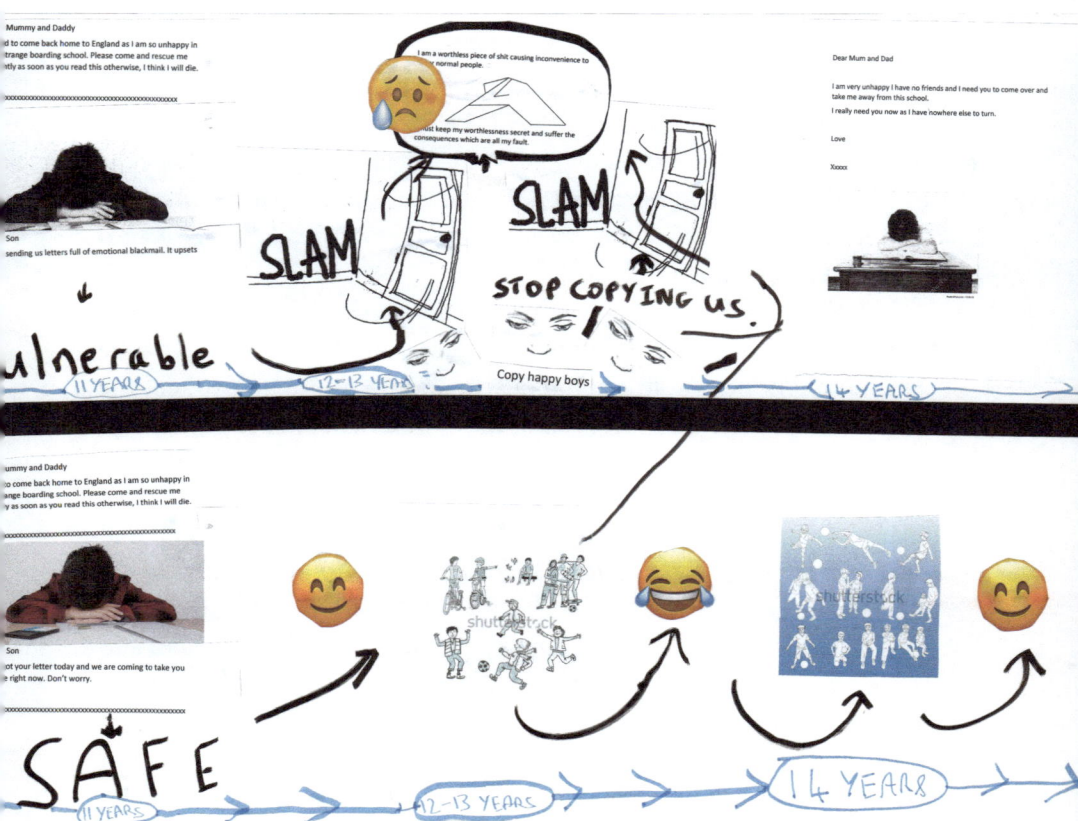

Panel 3: years 11–14

that extraordinary, but true: these were very hard habits to break. He was nearly sixty, in his office and yet part of him was still sitting on a bench, or waiting in a cot. Waiting to do things for other people. He felt guilty for having neglected Meg. He stopped and went downstairs.

When he took breaks, he worried that he would lose his momentum, that he would vanish from the beachhead and the sea would swallow his pathetic saga up. But he had to take breaks.

Sometimes it was difficult to get back to it.

He thought perhaps it wasn't something to be finished, not in an ordinary sense, but that working on it was how he could practise and build up new habits. It wasn't simple work. He didn't do it all in one go, he had to put it to one side and then go back to it again and again. That was how to build this app, it was a matter of practise. Practise was the app.

In the lower tier children went to school, got the right kind of attention. In the upper tier he was alone. He had gone through the motions of living but he'd done so as an outcast. He was always trying to copy the other children around him. He'd practised that enough. He could not be spontaneous, he had become false to himself and to everyone else, he'd become William the Emulator.

He told Julian about the work he was doing, showed him the panels as he worked on them. Julian encouraged him to carry on. Now he was in action like a soldier on a beach, and the more he worked, the more it came back to him, linking up, spontaneously. He felt he was going somewhere, he wasn't being put in his place. He was snipping the hot-wire.

Like the time he was winded and thought it better that he go off and die alone rather than try to get help. He'd felt that asking for help would mean more trouble. Julian said that meant these problems were older than thirteen, older than when he used to emulate friends at school and try to fit in. Sitting there looking at the images and timelines William recognised that must be right.

He remembered, right from the start, how Julian was interested in the word 'emulate'. It irritated him then, but it was true, this was older than Ireland and boarding school. It was already going on at primary school. Before then. Had it really been going on that long? It struck him as ironic that he was still caught in the questions although the answers were drawn on the paper in front of him in colour and in black and white. He looked back at the first panel: the sunshine days, a trampoline, an infant him being soppy with his mother. It wasn't going on then. But it didn't take long to start.

And when he was excited about the packed lunches—he could still recall the sense of excitement to tell his mother when he got home. And all it did was to make her angry. He couldn't do anything to make it up to her. That's why he did chores, dried dishes, washed up, wrestled with the enormous hoover, and spent his pocket money on gifts for them. They thought he was funny and he'd liked that, he liked it when he made them happy. But then he was left making his own Marmite sandwiches, because his mother insisted he did. At lunchtime at school, his sandwiches, wrapped in horrible grease-proof paper, looking like so much shit on toilet paper. He was ashamed and ate them alone. Not like his friends who would go to heaven with their neat heavenly lunches. The thought of it all started to overpower him.

> In the Bayeux Tapestry a woman and her child flee from a burning house.

He put the glue and images down, just dropped what he was doing, went downstairs and drank. Drank for the rest of the week. Thought about chucking it in again.

> ... on the 14th October 1066, the morning of the battle, William is shown in full armour, soon to mount his horse. William's Norman cavalry gallops off to face Harold's English soldiers.

He began to draw the boarding school years, falling out with his friends, them telling him to stop copying them. Hiding himself away.

'Why are you always copying us? Eh?' The shame of it still cast a shadow across him. He fashioned images of the boy-him sending letters home for help, only to be rejected. Not rejected, crushed. He used the image of a door being slammed, he repeated it in different panels. His father came, sat him on a bench, said 'Don't send us anymore of these emotional blackmail letters'. The horror and shame of his own letter being waved in his face. He glanced round his office at the neat stacks of fine Italian paper tied up in blue ribbons, the envelopes on his shelf. He still wrote letters to his daughters. He liked fine handmade paper, he'd brought paper back from Amalfi for another project he'd never been able to pursue.

If he was better at drawing he would fit all of the images in, make it as long as the Bayeux Tapestry, he'd include an image of Stan running to catch the boys. He'd never seen anyone run like that. It scared him almost more than when the bullies chased them. Stan ran for his son, for both of them, arms pumping, he didn't want his son to be picked on, or his friend. Stan didn't want to teach his son a hell of a lesson, he wanted to teach the bullies a lesson. He remembered how guilty he felt that Stan was treating him as someone who had value. When he looked at it all on paper, laid out, drawn out, looked at the events on the pages like this, it became different. He tried to step back, survey it. Then, inspired by the

Bayeux Tapestry, he took care to stick the pages together so they formed one long set of images, a codex.

Drawing his timeline, he could see the story of himself, see the contexts of his problems laid out. Looking at it gave him perspective, it did help him to step back from obsessing about it all of the time. He could see how it had been going on all these years. There were moments when he got a break from it, when he stopped being someone waiting in a bedroom, in a cot, waiting to be rescued from school. When he focused on the drawing it helped. When he worked on it there was no hyperarousal, no fear of being put in his place. It was like when he watched David Bellamy's programmes, being able to get lost in David Bellamy's enthusiasm, his passion, being down in the weeds crawling after newts with him. That's what he wanted, to take all of this passion into his projects and ideas. He laughed to himself in his office with the papers looping over his lap and onto the floor. With a Pritt stick in one hand and a picture of a gin bottle stuck to the fingers of the other. Right now he could remember; it wasn't that there were things wrong with him, it was that things had happened to him.

Still, when Meg or one of the girls came into the house the instinct to conceal it, to put other people first, nearly overpowered him. He felt it move through him in a rush, through his heart and skin and up to his scalp. The vigour of it. The hot-wire. Stress hormones need time to be metabolised—he had discussed that with Julian. It might be like a kind of post-traumatic symptom: you didn't stop it, but you could learn to live with it. To metabolise it. Gradually he felt himself settle, stability returned. First he had to settle, reset himself, then he could come back to the images, to concentration and to flow. He left the images spread out where they were across his desk, across the floor.

With care, he drew the priest touching him, the right hand snaking under bedsheets. Grooming?

'I think you were groomed,' said Julian. He was having none of it. But then uncannily, grooming cases started to appear in the news: Savile, then Andy Woodward's book, a boy who wanted to play football, and Paul Bennell, a coach who knew that made Woodward vulnerable because it was something to exploit. Woodward said Bennell groomed his whole family. William could see that when someone knows you need

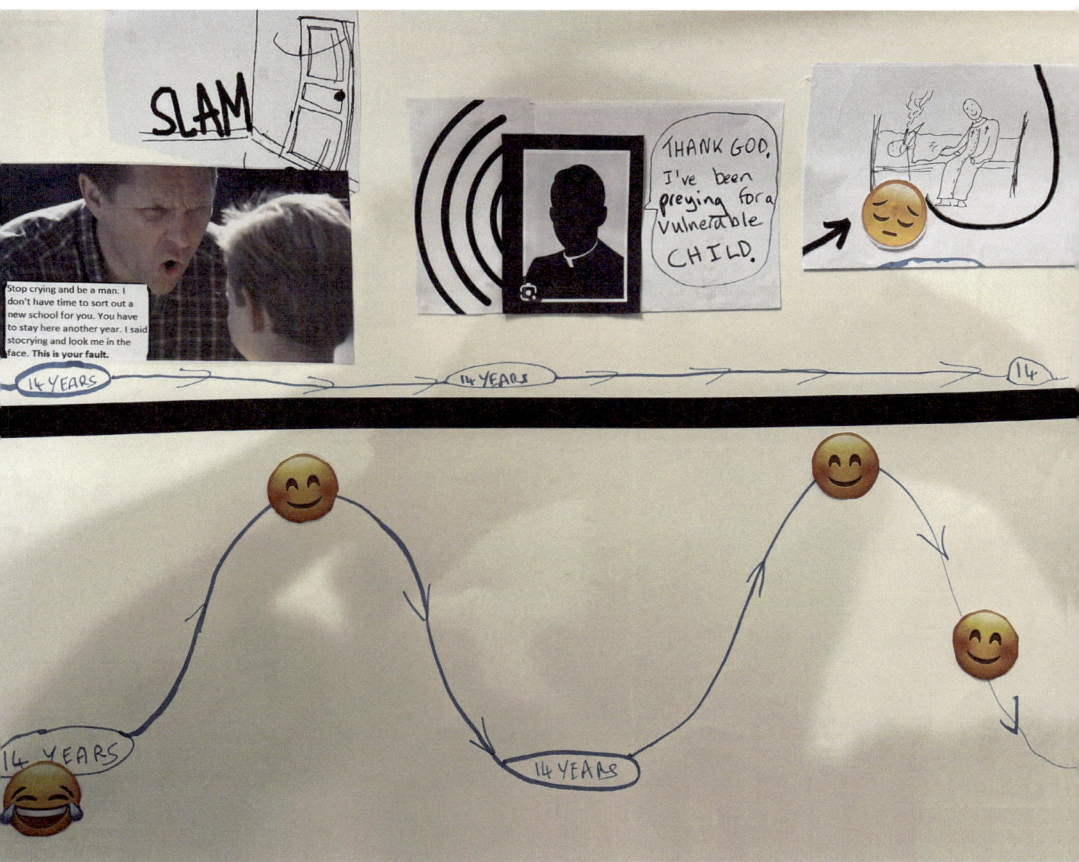

Panel 4: year 14

something you can be exploited while all the time being made to think it's you that's responsible. And that's what grooming is. He'd like to tell people about the true nature of grooming. What image could he use for the priest? He Googled his school, found their website, explored it and discovered that the priest had died. He sat looking at the obituary, puzzling over it.

In the Bayeux Tapestry a lookout warns Harold of the approaching Norman army.

William drew eyes, his own eyes looking down from his place at everyone else in humanity below. He glued the door being slammed on him again.

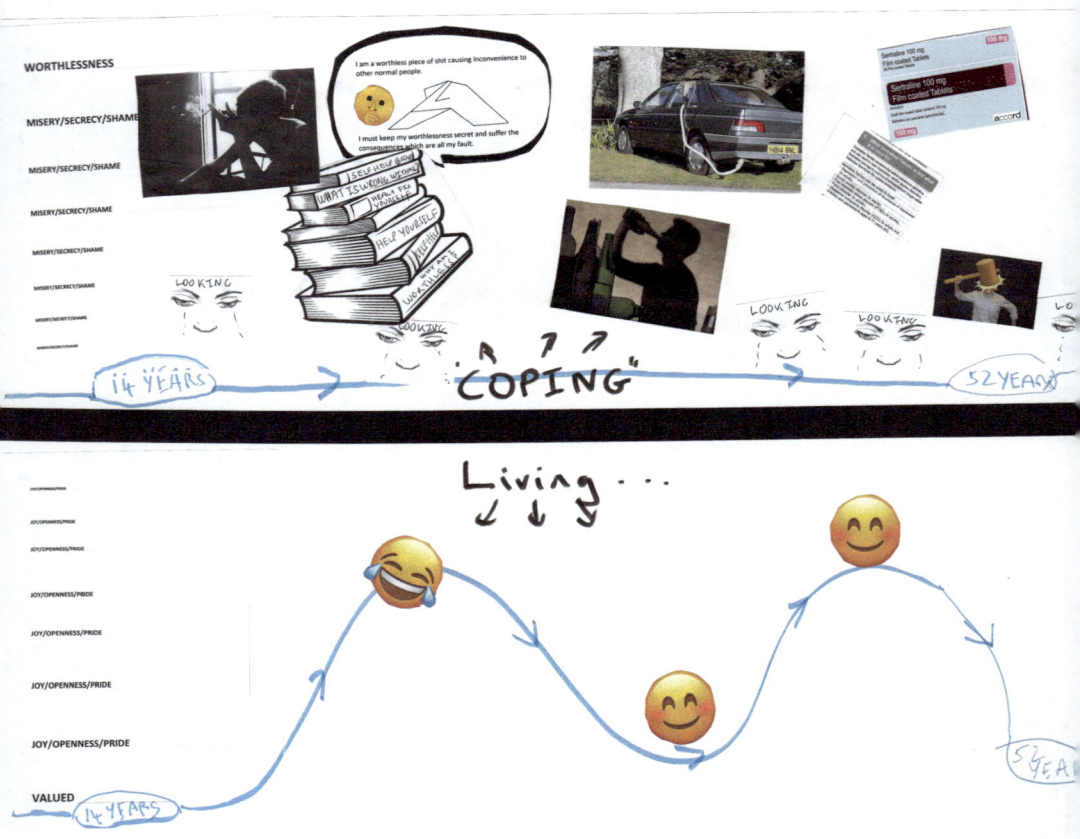

Panel 5: years 14–52

Grooming? He only wanted tobacco. The priest used that to groom him? Yes, that was the right word, so he would use it. He was vulnerable, like Woodward, like all vulnerable people, like all the girls in Bradford who still say the men who abused them were good to them. Jimmy Savile, *Jim'll Fix It*. He could see it then: if ever there was a television show designed by a groomer. 'Tell me what you want and I'll fix it for you.' That was the essence of grooming.

Then life after school, coping? Coping? Working, taking himself away to find himself, drinking, having seizures in the South Pacific. The fear that others would see how little he valued himself. A suicide attempt, meeting with a hypnotherapist. Now he fit all of these images into the story: the über mallet, the silhouette of the man glugging from the bottle. Laying it all out in this timeline, watching

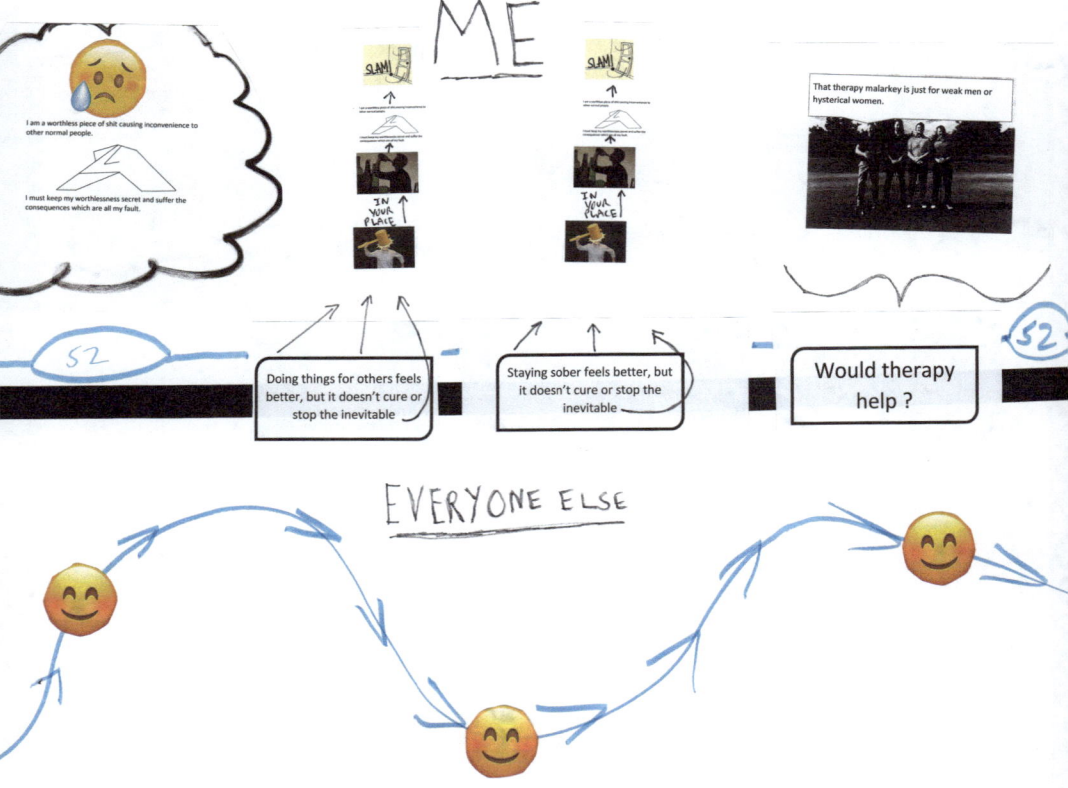

Panel 6: me and everyone else

the pages extend, coming out, his codex, his paper app. He could see himself in it.

But his eyes were feeling the strain, he adjusted the angle poise. Rested, leant back in his chair. He could see this wasn't a fairy tale, that pitfalls remained. If something went wrong in his work, his mood might dip. He might not remember the event that triggered it. That was the thing about it, you didn't remember that something had happened to you, you just presumed there was something wrong with you. He didn't remember the contexts. That was the point of the images, trying to create a personal aide-memoire, a short-cut way of reminding himself who he was, what he had been through, his history, his contexts.

He took images to the sessions and laid them out on the floor in Julian's garden room and they looked at them together. There was more and more of it, all these different versions. William liked the idea

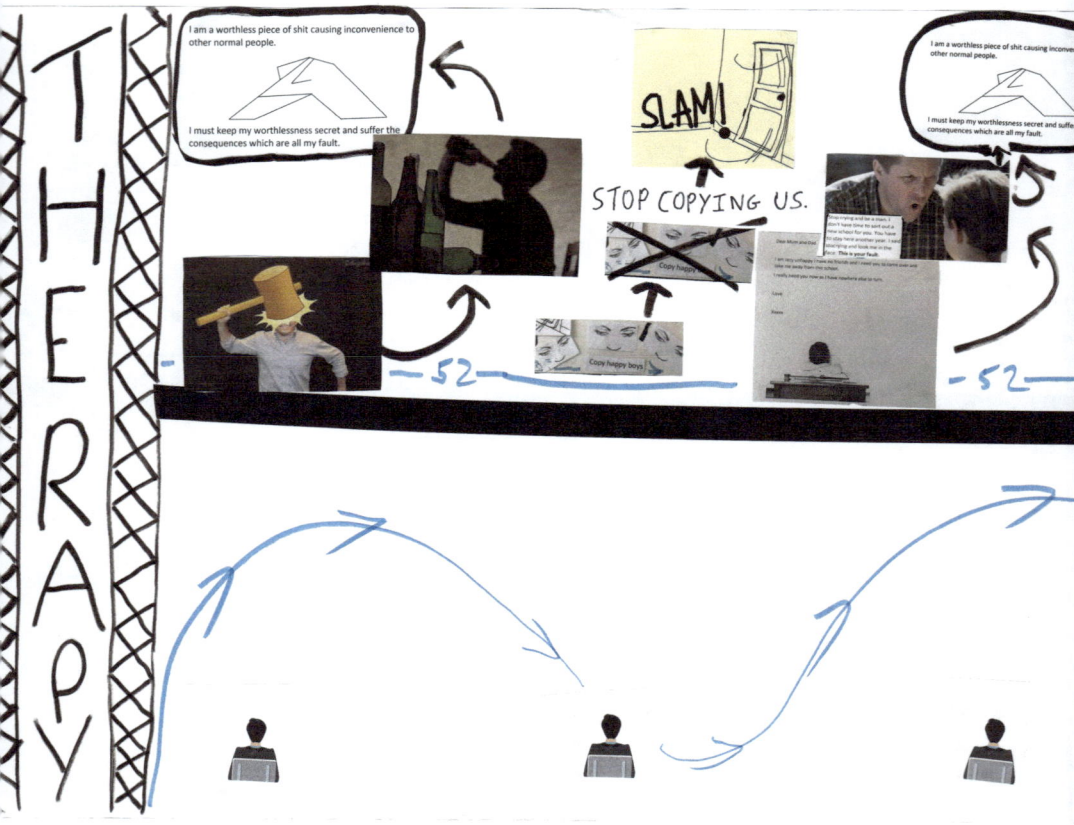

Panel 7: therapy #1

of it forming a codex, like the Bayeux Tapestry. Julian liked the idea of William reminding himself of his history, his contexts, meeting his demons, not once and for all, but again and again.

William wanted a conclusion. If there were all of these panels describing trauma and its after-effects, then William wanted to include an image that represented the achievement of health and stability, some better alternative, but he couldn't find it. Not in a meaningful or enduring way. For Julian, a conclusion would be a work in progress, not a fixed outcome, but a way to be able to reflect on himself and how he was living. A way to remember, a way to develop a sanctuary of his own.

Julian said that after trauma things were different, you weren't the person you were before it, William could see that was true. There was his line dividing the page of himself, not like it was before though—it was more permeable now.

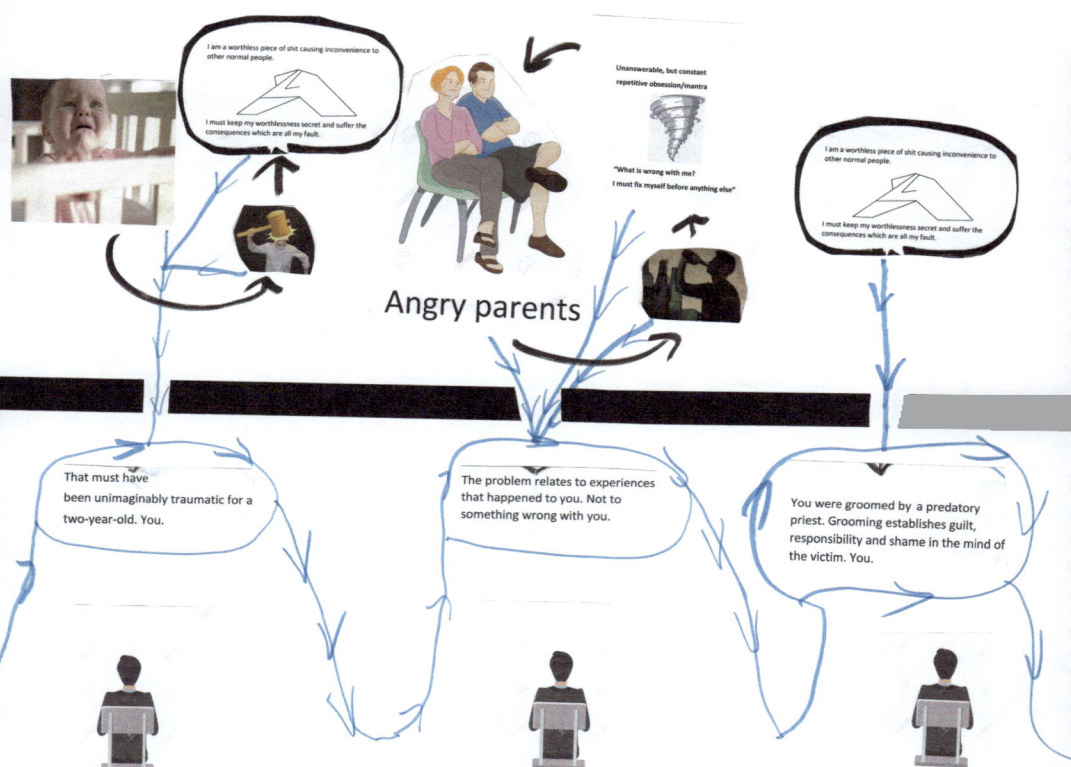

Panel 8: therapy #2

Sometimes there were breaks and William was with the rest of humanity. Then there was greater stability.

He was William and Harold facing himself on the beach, holding a measured truce.

This was different to what the nuns had stitched. Peace on the beach, a different outcome?

The early morning worthlessness had stopped.

He hadn't killed himself.

He had stayed married.

He had cut down his drinking.

He had cut down the flipping.

He had stopped telling himself he was a worthless piece of shit.

He was even able to enjoy a beach holiday.

And when a flight was delayed, he didn't think it was his fault—well not always.

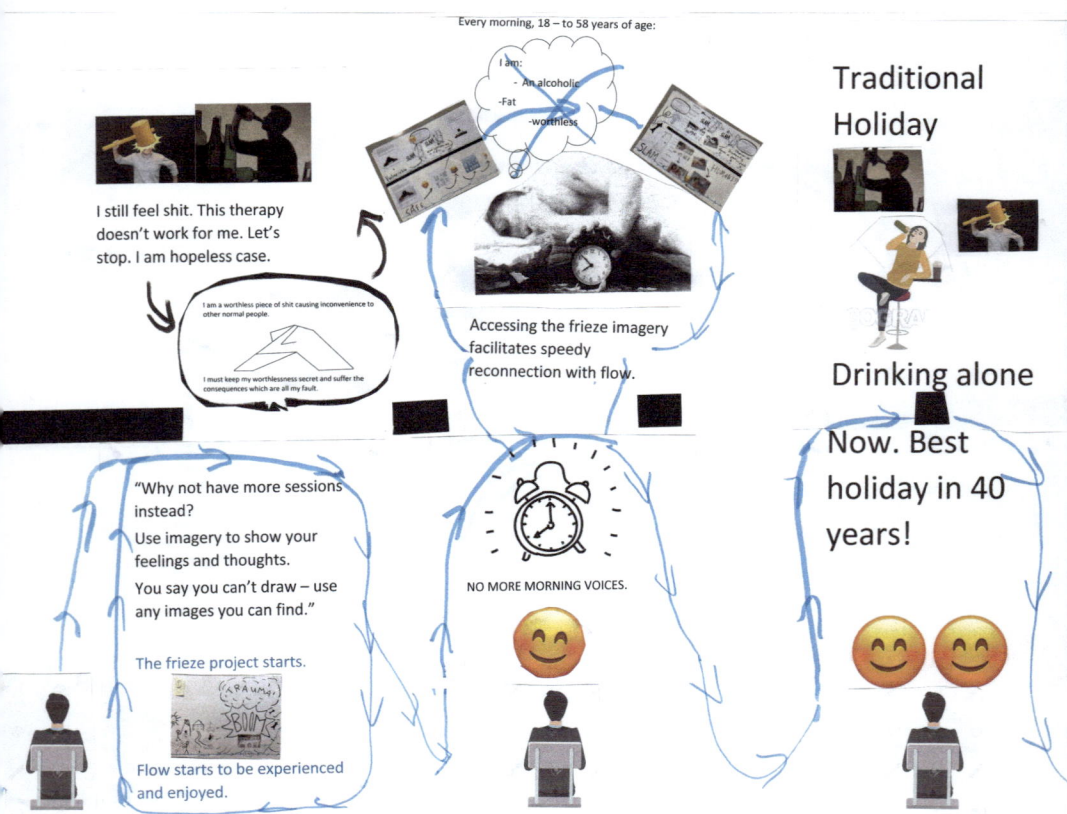

Every morning, 18 – to 58 years of age:

I am:
- An alcoholic
- Fat
- worthless

Accessing the frieze imagery facilitates speedy reconnection with flow.

I still feel shit. This therapy doesn't work for me. Let's stop. I am hopeless case.

I am a worthless piece of shit causing inconvenience to other normal people.

I must keep my worthlessness secret and suffer the consequences which are all my fault.

"Why not have more sessions instead?
Use imagery to show your feelings and thoughts.
You say you can't draw – use any images you can find."

The frieze project starts.

Flow starts to be experienced and enjoyed.

NO MORE MORNING VOICES.

Traditional Holiday

Drinking alone

Now. Best holiday in 40 years!

Panel 9: therapy #3

Part VI

Coming out

Chapter 22

William waited while the printer, an elegant middle-aged woman, placed the slim stack of A4 paper on the counter and swept it flat with the palms of her hands. She looked at William from behind round glasses which she removed and set down on the counter between them.

'I have printed the two sets,' she said. William thanked her. Here he was, at the printers, collecting his images. Him and his Bayeux Tapestry out in the world. He wanted to pinch himself to check he wasn't dreaming.

The images had become too difficult to manage. There were so many parts to them: separate cut-out shapes, pictures, and stuck-down details. Each time he moved them, bits fell off that he struggled to reattach. He had made them on oversized paper, size AO. Then, inspiration came to him. He should find a printer who could reduce them to a more manageable size. That would mean taking them out into the world. He took detailed pictures, emailed them, and now here he was.

The printer nodded to herself. She looked like she was trying to find the right way to say something. She drew a breath and held it for a moment.

'If you don't mind me saying so, I found them rather moving,' she said. William was surprised. At first, he had an impulse to shut her comment down, to ask for the bill and leave, but then just as quickly, it passed, and he realised he didn't mind her saying so. He gave a smile, aware that he felt rather moved too.

'No, not at all,' said William. 'Not at all.' He wondered if she could hear the emotion in his voice.

'They're very involving pictures. I think people would relate to them. I printed them last night and found myself thinking of them through the evening. They're ... well they're engaging, relatable.'

'Rather rough I think,' said William.

'No. Well, that might be part of the appeal, part of why people would relate to them. They made rather an impression on me. There's something about them.' With care she tapped the papers together, squared them off, and placed them in a large brown envelope. She paused then, looked down, placed her hand on her glasses and then turned back to him.

'But I do have one question ... did they catch him?' She looked down at the envelope, then back at William.

William, surprised, looked across at her open face. He could see she really had thought about it. He wasn't sure what to say, he hadn't expected this. She gave him a brief worried smile. He scratched his right ear, then found his voice again.

'No,' said William, 'in fact he died before anything could happen.'

'Ah,' she said, her expression softened. 'I wondered. I'm glad you brought them here.'

Then he was aware of an urge to ask her lots of questions about what she liked? What she found interesting? What she thought about it all? He was full of questions. Not that she'd have known it by his silence. He pressed his fingertips against the edge of the countertop. He hadn't expected this. Here he was, out in the world with his pictures, at the printers, having a conversation about them.

Then she turned, went to the till, rang up the bill and returned to give it to William who stood, waiting, still wondering at her reaction, her question, his questions.

He took out his wallet and paid.

'Thank you,' said William.

'Thank you,' she said.

Chapter 23

'I bring images,' said William holding the brown envelope in his hand. He set it down on the pale rug in front of him, swivelled his chair and placed his keys and glasses on the inlaid table.

'I see,' I said.

'Yep.' William looked down at the envelope and then looked up, an arched, inquisitive expression on his face. 'Do you want to see them?' I smiled, nodded.

'Yes.'

'Good.' He started to remove the papers from the envelope. I saw the care he took as he did so. 'They're not going to fit on your desk. I had two copies printed, one's for you.' He started to separate the papers into two piles, then stopped. 'And do you know what?' William paused for effect. I didn't, I waited for him to continue. 'We've had our first review.' I wasn't sure what to make of the comment, I looked over my glasses at William. 'I got these sets made at my local printers. When I collected them the manager asked if she could talk to me about them. I was surprised, a bit concerned, thought I might be in trouble. At first I thought not to, but then I realised that I didn't mind her asking, didn't even mind answering her questions. She said how interesting she thought they were, and that people would relate to them, that she related to them. I could see she'd really thought about them. I was touched by her interest.' William had now separated the images, he sat back in his chair, looked at me. 'Then, and I didn't see this coming either. She asked if they'd caught him?' He lowered his head, reached down, picked up the envelope and placed it on the throw folded at the foot of the couch.

I uncrossed my legs and turned a few degrees in my chair. I hadn't seen that coming either.

'Right,' I said, 'that is interesting.' I thought of William being able to show his images to people, to talk about them, I thought that was remarkable in itself.

William looked up, the printed pages in his hand.

'I'm not sure where to put these? I'd like you to see them in sequence.'

'Could we spread them out on the floor?' I asked.

William nodded.

'Yes, I think we could.'

With that, William began laying the papers out between us. I saw they were numbered.

'They fit together?'

'Yes, they make a codex. I meant to tape them together but ran out of time.'

'Right', I said. William scanned the floorspace.

'I'm not sure if they'll fit in here,' said William. 'And I had them reduced from the originals I'd made, that's why I was at the printers. I may still do more on them.'

We laid the A4 sheets out together, taking care to match up the edges as best we could. We had to move the chairs to make space. I could see the images linked chronologically from William's earliest memories of childhood to now.

'This first panel is from nought to two years,' said William. 'The images on the left of it are me with my family before the disasters, pre traumas. Then boom, here,' he pointed to an explosion, 'it all goes wrong. I am put up in my cot and left there. The door is slammed on me. That's when everything changed. That's why the rest of the images are divided into two. The upper tier, that's me in my worthless place. The lower tier, that's everyone else in humanity.' I looked at the panels, taking them in.

'It's quite something, seeing it laid out like this,' I said.

'Yes,' William continued to adjust and position them, he gestured. 'It's my own Bayeux Tapestry. And that's school, the priest, grooming. This is the coping panel, and this is when I started coming to see you. That's you in the lower tier looking at me.' I saw the image of myself. William sat back on the edge of his chair, thinking. 'I'd like to do something with it,' said William.

'What sort of a thing?'

'I'd like to put it in a huge frame and send it to the Royal Academy for the Summer Exhibition.' I thought that would be something. 'I showed some of the panels to Meg, I'm not sure what she made of it, but I know it helped me to show her. It was me telling my story, coming out. Like speaking with the printer, I want to tell more people about this.' William leant forward and adjusted two of the images.

I looked from one detail to another. I thought the door slams worked very well, dynamic. Thought so much of it worked well. I found it remarkable how William had developed it, how he'd told the story. And the scale of it. I could imagine the printer was interested.

'Telling my story, that's the opposite of waiting in my cot for my mother or father to come and rescue me and make everything better,' said William. I looked back at the first and second panel. 'It's the opposite of being stuck in an obsessional loop. That's where I've always gone when I have time on my hands. I wait to be rescued, and I do things for other people. Buy presents for my parents with my pocket money. I emulate. You picked up on that at the start, emulation. Where had I learned to emulate? Do you remember how you asked about that?'

'I do.'

'That stayed with me,' said William. I looked at him. Sunlight that had been warming the edge of the window frame now fell on the pale rug, drawn as it were, to discover the images with us. 'But, I'll tell you what I think should be done with this.' He paused, looking at me. 'I think it should be a book. Each image should be laid out, and there should be text to explain it. I think you should write the text.'

'Right,' I said, leaning back, thinking William's idea over. I hadn't seen that coming. I wondered if it would be appropriate. 'That might be a bit unorthodox,' I said taking off my glasses.

'How so?'

'Well, I'm not sure, but people might wonder if I had got you to do something for me. If I had got you to spend your pocket money on me, so to speak, something like that.' William frowned at the idea, glanced out of the window at the olive tree, then back to me.

'Well they might,' he said, 'but there's more to it than that. It's telling the story, breaking the silence, the weight of the shame. You could write about how people are spotted and groomed, how I was spotted and groomed. Write words that might help people understand more about what grooming is, what trauma is. Words that teachers, policemen, everyone could read. Words that would help vulnerable people, help them before predators get them.' William broke off there, leant forward and with care lined up panels three and four as best he could. He sat back in his chair, swept his hand through his thinning hair. 'Not that I think this is all about grooming. But I think drawings like this would make sense to people. It made sense to the printer. I didn't expect that. She said she thought people would relate to them. It might even encourage other people to draw their own images, timelines, might help them understand what's happened to them. Help them understand why they get stuck in obsessional loops. How to stop going down rabbit holes. People can say what they like about this. The fact is that doing this has helped me change the way I feel about myself. I don't think I am to blame for everything anymore. That's a good thing. And I'm not drinking so much, Meg has noticed that. That's a good thing. I can concentrate more on me and my things now. That's a good thing. People can say what they want, but this is a good thing.' He looked down at the printed images and back to me. 'I was able to have this printed, to come out, to let a stranger see it. I never would have been able to do that.' He looked at me. 'I think I'm complimenting you, myself. Both of us. That's a good thing too.'

I looked at the panels, thinking over his comments and ideas. I could see that a lot of people might benefit from drawing their own timelines.

'The image there, that's a stand-in for the priest?' I said.

William looked down.

'Yes. It is. I was thinking of using some image from a horror film for him. Bela Lugosi, Boris Karloff. Then I thought, what have they ever done to me? I thought I should use that image. I went to the school website and looked him up, it turned out he died a while ago. I found his obituary too. I wondered about including that. I'm thinking of contacting the school, telling them about him, asking them to remove him from their website, seeing as I won't get my day in court.' William reached back to the envelope, retrieved a folded piece of paper and handed it to me. I put my glasses back on and saw I was holding a copy of the priest's obituary.

'It says he adored children and worked tirelessly at ********? What's ********?' I said, looking up, lowering the page. William stared back at me, blank.

'I'm not sure.'

'You didn't Google it?'

'No,' said William, surprised he hadn't. He looked at me. 'I don't know why I didn't, I've been rushing around, could you? Now I mean? I don't have my phone.' I picked up my phone and typed into the search bar.

'I see,' I said. The results were full of abuse allegations.

'See what?' said William. I looked up, took a breath, then read from the phone.

'******** was an orphanage, in ********' I stopped, looked at William. 'Here look' I handed William my phone. William took it, sat back reading, while the sunlight moved onto the images on the floor.

'That's where the priest must have come from,' said William, lowering the phone. 'God, it's like something from the child abuse inquiry.' I nodded. I thought that too. He looked at the phone again, then leant forward and handed it back.

———•———

Later that evening, my mind returned to the conversation with William, I couldn't concentrate on anything else. I decided to go for a walk.

Leaving my house I walked down a bridleway and crossed onto a wide farm track that ran through ripening wheat fields. I came to a point where the path turned to run along the bank of the river Thame. I thought of William at school, out searching on lanes for cigarettes and red-top matches. Then smoking by himself. Standing in his Paradise Woods, leaning, in the dark, alone against a tree. I pictured a cigarette end flicked on an arc towards the river, dying out as it floated away on a slow current like this one.

I'd often wondered if we would be able to get to the end of our work together. I thought of all of the work I'd been involved with that had broken off prematurely. All of the people who had abandoned therapy with me, who had suddenly been discouraged by something I said or one thing or another. People who had been distracted and lost their momentum, lost their confidence. People who settled for a break in their mood rather than following the impulse that had brought them further. William was different, he'd stuck at it. I hadn't seen this coming. Is that where we were? Approaching the end?

And the pictures. I was impressed by the pictures. How they grew from each other, fitted together. A codex?

Now when we met, the floor was covered with the images William created and built up. And the fact that William had taken it to the printers, broken his cycle of isolation, had let himself come out. And as we spoke about them, William edited them. When he returned the next time, they were changed. It was now over nine metres long. I wondered what the Royal Academy would make if a frame that size turned up. I liked that idea. I'd like to paste the images up as a frieze around my walls.

I could see that the moment I suggested we both went to the desk and began looking at the images together, that moment, that spontaneous moment, was a point we had both worked to arrive at, a kind of turning point. I wondered if all the time we'd spent together had led to that benign moment. A moment where defences were relinquished? The end of a battle? Trust between us, trust internalised, a benign therapeutic moment. I'd once meant to write something about that. William had come to feel confident enough to trust himself, to come out, to snip the hot-wire. I found that very moving.

I stood in the fading light, in the dusk on the riverbank, amid the insects and the dust and felt a sense of gratitude. Gratitude, to have been able to be part of this work, to get to this point together, a privilege I'd never imagined. The intimate sense of trust between us. We'd recovered William's capacity to trust and to concentrate. It was remarkable.

And now, William thought I should write a book to go with the pictures, his codex, a story that would reveal the depth of the images. I wasn't sure about it, could I even do it? I liked the idea of being able to tell people about the work. Was it the right thing to do? William didn't think these kinds of questions came into it.

———•———

'This should be a book,' said William. 'I think other people would relate to it.' He stopped, waiting for me to respond.

'No?' said William. 'I'm not hiding away, not worthless, not shamed. I'm not drinking in secret, well hardly, certainly a lot less. This is coming out. This is telling a story. This is the opposite of grooming. People will relate to this, they might get something from it. Look how the printer did.'

I did think of that.

'What kind of a book are you thinking of?' I asked.

'A tale, like Oliver Sacks said, and it should include some of your ideas about trauma, grooming. But it should be your book,' said William, then added, 'maybe it would give you a chance to come out.'

I smiled. I wondered if there might be something in that.

———•———

Standing at the river's edge I thought the idea over. A tale, a book for ordinary people, not just for academics, therapists and counsellors. A tale for a reader. I liked that idea. A book that would keep William's story in the foreground. I didn't want to write an academic book, or a book about a therapist.

I imagined going to the Royal Academy, the pleasure of seeing William's images hanging on the wall. Maybe I could write words that William could include as footnotes to the images. Perhaps I'd start there.

Across from me an engine ripped into life, breaking my thoughts. I dragged my gaze up from the rivers' swirls and weeds. I made out a man on a sit-down mower starting to work his way around the lawn on the other side.

And it wasn't just trust that'd been recovered, it was William's capacity to concentrate. That fact held my attention. William could never concentrate, not on his own things. Now look at him. A codex, a book? I felt that my own concentration and trust had improved too. I had learnt more than what a codex was: now I understood more about what grooming was, how it worked. Could I write about trauma and grooming?

A number of high-profile grooming cases had come to light during our work, and inquiries into historic sexual abuse. Andy Woodward's book about grooming in football made a particular impression on William. And there was Savile, the arch groomer. The Bradford grooming gang, Epstein. There would be more people, they might be interested in William's story.

The question of what grooming is seemed to operate on the borders of personality and society. In a kind of non-place, a place where things cannot be properly known or spoken about, or kept in mind. The characteristics that victims display are obscure and paradoxical. The victim can't talk about what's happened. Grooming corrupts, stifles spontaneity and freedom of expression. Innocence is lost. I wondered if this might be to do with the way it was linked in some way with personal desire, with a corrupt sense of guilt and blame. The victim can't speak about it. The predator is insidious, they work like the priest by stealth to cultivate trust and indebtedness, to exploit the vulnerable person's unmet needs. It looks like the person is being given what they need, but that is a Trojan horse. In plain sight, the victim is being bent out of shape, attacked from within by shame, their potential and creativity ransacked. Silenced. And all the while the victims develop fierce loyalty to their groomers and are powerless to break the cycle. That was the grooming paradox. The victim goes back to the groomer when the groomer starts to give attention to someone else. This vindicates the groomer, that is the endgame. The abuser makes out they have done a service and the victim is racked with guilt.

I could see that it was a subject that was not easy to discuss. It was probably an ancient coercive form of human relationship. There was the strange way in which cases brought to court seemed destined to drift out of the public mind. There must be something about grooming, sexual abuse, and trauma that makes it hard to keep it in mind— the intensity of the shame. I could write something about that. Write something that might help prevent grooming relationships? Could it help educate? To make it simpler to identify vulnerable individuals, to help eliminate the culture of bullying, to strip the oxygen from the predator's world?

William's situation should have been spotted and addressed appropriately, his school grades suddenly sliding from As to Ds, his absence in the school sports teams. His perverse reactions to compliments. A book would give the chance to set some of these ideas out before readers.

I was uncertain about the idea of showing any text I wrote to William; it would be an unusual thing to do, but then again our work was unusual. What could I write about trauma? Could I show it, dramatise it? This work did make clear the way early trauma creates vulnerability, vulnerability that predators are tuned to spot.

Chapter 24

I handed William an A4 page, perhaps it could be a footnote to his images. There was a silence as he read. In the silence I found myself looking at the knots in the walls, then out of the window behind William. I detected William's aftershave. Was it cedar? Something dry? I'd never been sure.

> When trauma happens, particularly in very early life, it can be life-changing. One complication arises because the trauma occurs before the child has developed a secure sense of their position in the world. The child does not have a sufficiently secure sense of identity to fall back on.
>
> In a situation where there is no parent or adult available to help the child through what has happened, these experiences are incomprehensible. They cannot be assimilated like other things. This means that childhood trauma and breakdown can occur and remain experiences that are unacknowledged, but which nonetheless go on to undermine and influence the way future life develops. When there are repeated traumas, the effects are compounded.
>
> The child has no way of making sense of what has happened to them. So, they come up with their own explanation: the trauma

happened because of something they did, it was their fault. This is
the start of a new identity based on worthlessness. After trauma, you
are no longer the person you were; you carry the trauma, the shame,
the wounds within you without knowing it. This makes you vulnerable
to further traumas.

'That's right,' said William. 'I had to come up with a way of understanding my place in the world. Everyone else was normal. I could only copy and emulate people, my father, boys at school. I had no worth of my own. I was stuck in this secret sense of worthlessness. The rest of the world were in humanity, not me.' William leant forward, animated, pointing at the pictures on the floor. 'After I was two I was always in my place, there in the upper tier. These are the words I meant are needed to explain the images. They need this kind of explanation.'

He lifted the paper, carried on reading.

After trauma, this becomes the new starting point. Now the child
comes to assume a new identity formed from the experience of
being imprisoned in an inner world in which they are tyrannised by
feelings of worthlessness, blame, shame, and guilt. This, in turn, leaves
the child vulnerable to further emotional instability, breakdown,
and trauma.

'That should be in the book,' said William. 'A part of me, trapped in trauma, still wanting to live in a fairy tale where my mother came to my room to find me and console me, and then took me downstairs and we ate eggs and toast and were soppy together. That didn't happen. It's not going to happen. But I don't blame myself for wanting it to. It should all go in the book.'

I nodded. I still wondered what kind of book it could be. The story of our work, the images, would have to be part of it.

'The child does not have sufficient identity to fall back on, that's me, was me. I've always said if the trauma had happened to me when I was twenty-five, I might have had a sense of who I was before it. But I didn't. I didn't have, how did you put it?' He looked back at the printed words, '... a secure identity to fall back on.'

'Now it doesn't feel like that?' I said.

'No, I think it feels different now.' I nodded. William continued reading.

> Grooming is the name we give to the process whereby a vulnerable individual with unmet needs, such as appropriate care and protection, is identified and exploited, sexually or otherwise, by a predator. In grooming, the predator identifies and responds to the victim by giving the victim the things they are missing and need. These needs will vary. William's desire for cigarettes was something the priest exploited.
>
> It is an important part of the process because it sets up the idea that everything that happens does so because the victim wanted it to. Grooming establishes guilt, responsibility, and shame in the mind of the victim.
>
> As the grooming progresses, this guilt and shame make it hard for the victim to tell their story and be believed. It is insidious. It becomes difficult for the victim to believe that the predator has done anything wrong.
>
> Grooming creates a guilty victim. The abuse is hidden in the identity of the individual. They may become chaotic, exhibit destructive behaviours, fail at school. In time attention may be drawn to a current problem like addiction, but the earlier, more destructive problem of grooming and sexual abuse is often not acknowledged.

William lowered his glasses.

'Perfect, I don't mean to big you up, but that's perfect.'

'Well, good, but I did it with you,' I said.

'No, no, no, you wrote that. Perfect. I think those paragraphs should be printed in every staff room in every school in the country. In the world. Put those paragraphs in the book.' William picked the page and his glasses up again and re-read the paragraphs. He lowered them again. 'Perfect. That should be compulsory reading for teachers, police, judges, social workers, family lawyers, barristers, religious institutions, orphanages, children's homes. Every child activity centre from football camps to ballet schools.'

I could see that William had come to recognise the obsessional loops that he fell into. Before, once he was in one, there was no coming back. Now he could recognise what had happened, and he was better at getting himself out of them. He was distinguishing the different states and feelings. He could come first now, he could work on the images, make his own Bayeux Tapestry, pursue creative ideas. I thought again that if there was a book, it was important that it was about William, not me.

William was drinking less, exercising a bit more. He was taking better care of his appearance. His business was going well and now when he went on business trips he stayed in better accommodation, he put himself first. He was looking after himself. I had watched him develop a level of emotional stability, that was something worth writing about. There were changes at home, too. William was no longer the Cinderguy doing everything for everyone else.

'Well I am certainly doing less,' said William. He swivelled in his chair, smiled.

'I was thinking, that if we'd met thirty years ago, if I had come to you instead of that hypnotherapist, how different things might have been. I was doing everything I could to get out of the mess I was in, endlessly reading self-help books.' He leant back. 'Nothing ever helped then. Things are different now. We have changed them. But there are also limits to what I can change. I mean, I don't know, but I think I could have changed more. There are still moments when I flip, when I'm back in my place. I can recognise it now. I can recognise what's happened, recognise that I've gone into that suspended state, the obsessional loop. When I recognise it, it's comforting, it's mitigating. You put it right in your text; you're not what you were before trauma. But it's how you live with that. You're not the same. And maybe if trauma had happened to me later, when I was twenty-five, then I might remember more about who I was. Of course I'll never know. But now I have insight. It's the insight that helps. In the past I had nothing, I just battled with it on my own, always ending up further down the rabbit hole. Now there is insight which brings armaments with it. It doesn't take away the trauma. There might still be the low mood, but there isn't the old destructive drinking. I understand what's going on, why it all happens. There isn't that old brutal internal voice, the über mallet smashing me to pieces. I can retain a sense of stability.'

I thought William was right, there were limits.

'This isn't a fairy tale, this is real. Things are different for me now, perhaps not everything has changed, but a lot has. You need to write it, tell it as a tale, like Oliver Sacks said: not a case study but a tale.' William had always liked Oliver Sacks' idea that the way to do justice to the complex interactions of a psychotherapeutic relationship was to tell it as a tale, not as a case study.

———•———

Across the late summer evenings I walked the bridleway down to the farm tracks again and again. I seemed to find it easier to walk and think than to sit and write. I walked to the river, stood, listened to it.

By the trees on the riverbank, I thought about the way we had learned to work together. The tensions, the agreements and disagreements, the mistakes I had made, saying the wrong things at the wrong times. Saying things when I might just have said less or nothing. The times when William had thought about leaving but somehow didn't. Most of all, how much I felt enriched by the work.

In the dark, slow-moving river's patterns I tried to make out my own reflection, tried to reflect on what we had done together. How do you judge work like this? I could see that creating the images had been helpful, a way for William to keep the events of his life nearer the front of mind, a way of remembering the things that had happened, of the context of his moods. Images that he could refer to, like a compass. Would writing a book add to that? Was it the right thing to do? Would it help William? Would it be relevant to some other reader in the future? Someone who knew nothing about either of them, like the girl William once saw hiding away against the school wall.

In my experience you can't cure profound psychic wounds, but you can become clearer about them, learn to live with them better, understand yourself more. Out of that knowledge you can nurture better emotional stability. You can't remove the injuries, but you might learn to live with them, learn to relate to them and yourself more. Out of our work together, trust had developed, William's defences had been stood down, and in the settled truce that followed, William's creativity and concentration emerged. And the thing that seemed so particular about this was that when the moment of trust occurred, it was William's concentration that shaped a way out of the endless repetitions of failure and into this new experience of mutual work and creativity.

I liked the idea of being able to tell people about what we had managed to do. I could see a book might be part of that, and I could see we were coming to the end of our work together.

These ideas flowed through my mind as I stood by the river. Sometimes I was tempted to wade in, to see if it was deep enough to swim. There was a narrow beach on the other side. I wondered if I could find a way to get to it.

Part VII

Psychotherapy ends

Chapter 25

'I am thinking it might be time to stop coming to see you,' said William.

We sat, the idea suspended between us in the silence. William looked at me, waited. I looked back at him.

'I think I can see that too,' I said.

William nodded, smiled, then turned to look out of the window at the olive tree. We were both silent.

'If I stopped,' said William, 'I'd like to think I could contact you again in the future … if I wanted to?'

I nodded.

'Yes,' I said. I was pleased that William had thought about that.

'In a way, I don't think it will stop. I think what we've done together is always going to stay in my mind. But if you were able to write about it too, if I could read about our work in a book, I think that would be satisfying.'

'Yes,' I said. 'I am thinking that I will try to.'

'Good,' said William. 'Good.'

So we picked a date and began the countdown to the end.

'Right,' said William. 'I think it will be good to take a bit of time over it. It makes me think of crossing off the days till I could leave school.'

I nodded, it didn't seem a very happy association. William looked at the desk, at the window. He turned back to me.

'It's not like that. But it has been a while, longer than I thought. Coming here, I mean.' He leant back, swivelled his chair to the window again, silent. He looked at the linen curtains, the objects on my desk that he had never properly made out.

'If you don't mind my asking, why are you here? I mean what drew you to this?' said William.

'This?'

'This work.'

'Ah,' I said. I looked down at the back of my hand resting on the edge of the chair. I fished for time. How would I start to answer that question? How would I explain the threads of my own that I'd followed and pursued? Things that had resonances with some of William's stories. That I had followed them until they led me to here? I didn't want to make this about me. Perhaps that was a story for another time. I wanted to make sure we kept our focus on our work. I looked up. 'Do you have any thoughts about that?' I said.

William laughed.

'Do I have any thoughts? No. But it's unusual work. Good work. But unusual.'

I nodded.

We continued to meet.

We sat and scanned the walls for the figures William had found amongst the knots. William continued to talk about the images. Sometimes he brought them to show how they continued to change and develop.

'You used to wonder if this was a prison, if you'd end up stuck here,' I said.

'Yes. I did. But it turned out there was a way out.'

I smiled, nodded. I wondered if perhaps I was trapped in the room. I knew I would miss William. We sat together. William appeared to absorb the room, the place, the silence, the motes of dust that crossed the shafts of moving sunlight, the sounds of traffic, the birdsong.

The night before the final session I had a dream. In the dream I was standing in the Royal Academy at the Summer Exhibition. There were groups of people milling about, talking, looking at pictures, drinking, laughing. There were so many pictures, I couldn't take them all in. Then people were walking towards me, but not to me. They were walking past me. I turned to see where they were going. Then I saw William's pictures framed on the wall, all of the images in one chronological sequence. I gazed up at them. An elegant man leant in to me, breaking my concentration.

'Isn't it all rather rough?' asked the elegant man.

'I think that's part of the appeal,' said a middle-aged woman, chipping in. 'I find it rather moving.' I listened to them. I saw then that David Bellamy had come up beside me. I was surprised.

'I thought you were dead,' I said.

'Ah well,' said David Bellamy, 'there's a bit more to it than that.' The elegant man turned to me, raised his eyes.

'What do you think of it?' he said. 'I mean who is this for?' I opened my mouth to reply but then I woke up.

I lay in the dark, fragments of the scene still on my mind. I checked the time on my phone, drank some water and tried to pull the dream back into focus. I couldn't get back to it.

Chapter 26

'Well,' I said, glancing at the clock, 'it is time to stop.' I had said these five words so many times, but this was the last time I would say them to William. For a moment we both sat still, neither of us made to move. Then William leant forward, I did too. We stood, stepped across the pale rug towards each other and shook hands.

'Thank you,' said William.

'You're welcome.' We stood in the middle of the garden office shaking hands, smiling at one another. Then we let go.

William turned and gathered up his wallet, glasses, keys, and mobile phone. He looked at me again, looked like he might say something, but didn't. He held his hand up, palm towards me and then tapped his chest. I nodded. Then William turned and left the room, taking care that the linen curtain didn't catch in the door as he pulled it shut.

I heard William's car start and stepped back to watch as he drove away. The car rolled, slowly creeping across the gravel, the left indicator starting to flash; it paused at the gate.

In his car, William glanced in the rear-view mirror and caught sight of the drive and the garden room behind. Then his car slid forward, out of my view and into his own future. I leant on my desk, looked at the nine images piled in the centre. I heard William's comment—'We have had our first review.' I wondered about this illustrated book. What should I call it? Names would have to be changed.

I looked at William's empty chair. I looked at the walls. Only then did I reach across to the Van Gogh print, lift it down and place it by the door.

I thought of William's comment that he might come back. He'd see the picture had gone, he'd have something to say about that. I took my notebook from the left-hand drawer of the desk, looked at it and turned it over in my hands.

A noise above distracted me: it was one of the jackdaws landing on the roof. I waited, heard the second one join it, heard them chatter. Could I include the birds in the book? They were part of the place. What could I include? What would I aim at?

I'd aim at telling the story of William without becoming caught up in psychological jargon. I'd avoid terminology as much as I could and give longhand, dramatised descriptions of situations and problems instead. I'd aim at the sense that the more that could be understood of William's experience and the contexts of his problems, the more a reader could relate to him. But I wasn't quite sure where to begin. Could I build it around William's images? Could I convey a sense of how our working relationship developed? I felt dubious about the whole idea.

Fragments from our conversations returned to my mind, jogging me. I sat, thinking, looking past the empty chair, aware of the murmur of traffic outside.

Perhaps I could start with William driving to meet me for the first time?